LOSE WEIGHT, LIVE WELL

"A Practical Guide to Achieving Your Weight Loss Goals
with Motivation, Nutrition, Exercise, and Tips"

*Transform Your Body and Mind
for a Healthier Life*

By

Dr. Murali Dama

This book is dedicated to all my supporters and family who have believed in me and encouraged me along the way. Without their love and support, this book would not have been possible. Additionally, this book is dedicated to all those who are currently on their own journey to transform their bodies and live a healthier and happier life. I hope that the information and tips shared in this book will serve as a valuable resource on your journey towards wellness.

CONTENTS

1. INTRODUCTION

Congratulations on purchasing this book! If you're looking for a comprehensive guide to help you lose weight and get in shape, then you've come to the right place. Are you ready to take control of your health and fitness? Losing weight and getting fit can be difficult and overwhelming, but it doesn't have to be. With the right plan in place, you can get the body you've always wanted and start living a healthier, happier lifestyle.

This book provides you with motivation, diet plans, workout tips, and other valuable information to help you reach your goals. You'll learn how to set realistic, achievable fitness goals, evaluate and select the right diet for you, and design your own effective workout plan. With this book, you can finally take control of your body and start transforming it into the shape you've always wanted. Weight-loss can be a challenging journey, and so many of us struggle to find the motivation and knowledge to start, stick to, and finish such a goal.

This book provides you with the tools and guidance you need to take charge of your health and make the weight-loss journey a manageable and successful one. Within the pages of this book, you'll find diet plans, workout regimens, and tips for getting the most out of every exercise and meal. We understand that everyone is unique and therefore, we provide you with the flexibility to create a plan tailored to your lifestyle and reach your health goals in no time.

One of the first steps in any weight loss journey is goal-setting.

It's important to set realistic and achievable goals that align with your overall health and fitness objectives. We will guide you through the process of setting goals and help you to stay motivated as you work towards achieving them.

Nutrition plays a critical role in weight loss and overall health. In this book, we will provide you with information on the different types of diets, such as low-carb, high-protein, and balanced diets. We'll also give you guidance on how to make healthy eating choices so that you'll be able to stick to your diet and reach your weight loss goals. Additionally, we'll provide you with tips on how to plan meals and snacks that are both healthy and satisfying.

Exercise is an important component of any weight loss journey. We'll provide you with a variety of workout plans, including strength training and cardio, to help you burn calories and build muscle. Additionally, we'll give you tips on how to get the most out of your workouts, such as proper form, intensity, and recovery.

Finally, we understand that weight loss is a journey and it can be challenging to stay motivated. That's why we've included tips and strategies to help you stay on track and achieve your goals. Whether it's finding an accountability partner, tracking your progress, or celebrating small wins, we'll provide you with the tools and support you need to stay motivated and achieve your weight loss goals. Don't wait any longer to start your weight-loss journey!

With the help of this book, you can create a plan that works for you and start seeing results. It's time to take charge of your health and start making the changes you need to reach your goals. This book is your guide to a healthier, happier, and more confident you. So, let's get started!

2. PROBLEMS WITH OVERWEIGHT

Weight management is an important aspect of overall health and well-being. Maintaining a healthy weight can help prevent a variety of health problems and improve overall quality of life. However, many people struggle with being overweight or obese, which can lead to a host of health issues. One way to determine if you are in a healthy weight range is by calculating your Body Mass Index (BMI).

What Is Bmi?

BMI is a measure of body fat based on height and weight. It is calculated by dividing a person's weight in kilograms by their height in meters squared, or by using a BMI calculator. The resulting number is then placed into one of several categories to determine if a person is underweight, normal weight, overweight, or obese. A BMI of 18.5-24.9 is considered normal weight, 25-29.9 is considered overweight, and 30 or higher is considered obese.

How To Calculate Your Bmi

Calculating your BMI is a simple process. You can use the formula:
BMI = Weight (kg) / [(Height(m)]2 or

BMI = 703 x Weight (lbs) / [(Height(in)]^2

use a BMI calculator like https://www.nhlbi.nih.gov/health/educational/lose_wt/BMI/bmicalc.htm.

It is important to note that BMI is not always a perfect indicator of health, as it does not take into account factors such as muscle mass or overall body composition. However, it is a useful tool for determining if a person is in a healthy weight range.

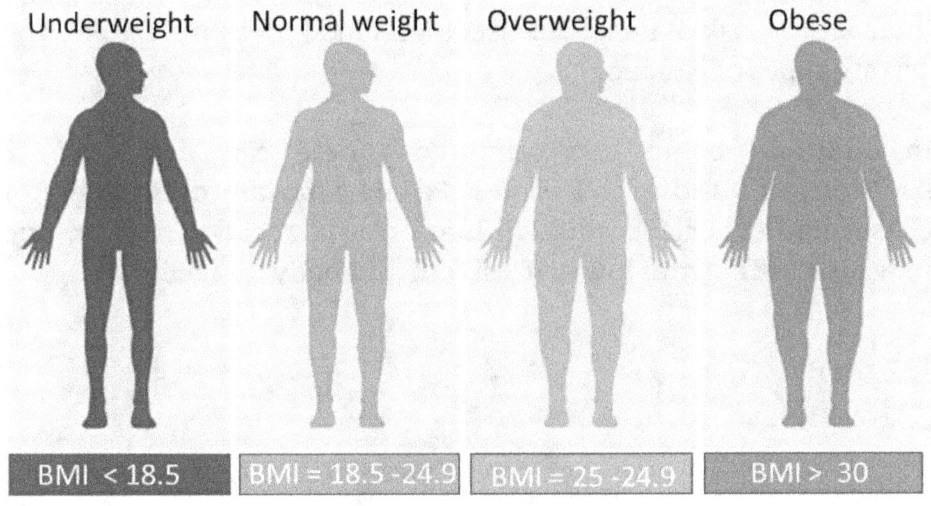

What are the optimum BMI levels?

BMI Categories:

Under Weight < 18.5

Normal weight = 18.5 – 24.9

Overweight = 25 – 29.9

Obesity > 30

Risks Of Being Overweight Or Obese:

Being overweight or obese can lead to a variety of health problems. One of the most common is type 2 diabetes. According to the World Health Organization (WHO), 87% of adults with diabetes are overweight or obese. Being overweight or obese can also increase the risk of heart disease, high blood pressure, stroke, and certain types of cancer.

In addition, being overweight or obese can also lead to psychological and social issues. People who are overweight or obese may experience discrimination and social isolation, and may also suffer from low self-esteem and body image issues.

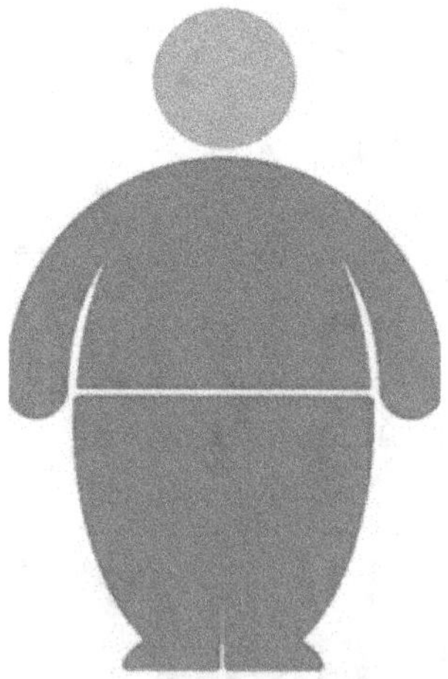

According to WHO global estimates data (from 2016), 1.9 billion adults (over age 18) are overweight and 650 million adults of these people are obese. Also estimates that approximately 40% of world population are overweight and about 13% of adult population are obese. More than 340 million children aged between 5-19 are obese or overweight now and more than 38 million children aged below 5 are overweight / obese.

Obesity and overweight are major public health issues that affect people of all ages. According to the World Health Organization, more than 1.9 billion adults were overweight or obese in 2016, and the prevalence of obesity has nearly tripled since 1975. Being overweight or obese increases the risk of developing several chronic diseases, including type 2 diabetes, heart disease, hypertension, and stroke.

There are several causes of obesity and overweight, including poor diet, lack of physical activity, and genetics. A poor diet high in calories and low in nutrients can lead to weight gain and obesity. Eating junk food, processed food, and large amounts of carbohydrates can prevent the body from getting the nutrients it needs, leading to weight gain. Additionally, eating large quantities of food can lead to overeating, which can cause weight gain.

Genetics also play a role in overweight and obesity. Genes can make people more likely to be overweight or obese, and some people may have a greater risk of developing certain conditions related to obesity. For example, people with a strong family history of type 2 diabetes may be more likely to develop the condition if they are overweight or obese.

The health risks associated with obesity and overweight are numerous. People who are overweight or obese are at an increased risk of developing several chronic conditions, including type 2 diabetes, heart disease, and stroke. Additionally, being overweight or obese can lead to joint pain, depression, and other psychological issues.

The best way to prevent or treat obesity and overweight is to make long-term, sustainable lifestyle changes. This includes eating a healthy, balanced diet, engaging in regular physical activity, and limiting unhealthy foods. Additionally, people should strive to maintain a healthy weight by controlling portion sizes, eating slowly, and limiting snacking.

In conclusion, obesity and overweight are serious public health issues that can lead to a variety of chronic conditions. Making long-term lifestyle changes, such as eating a healthy diet and engaging in regular physical activity, is the best way to prevent or treat obesity and overweight. Additionally, people should strive to maintain a healthy weight by controlling portion sizes, eating slowly, and limiting snacking.

Causes Of Overweight And Obesity:

There are several causes of overweight and obesity. The most common causes are unhealthy diet and lack of physical activity.

Unhealthy Diet: Consuming foods high in sugar, saturated fats, or trans fats, and low in fiber can contribute to weight gain and obesity. Processed foods, fast foods, and sugary drinks are also considered unhealthy and can lead to weight gain. High-fat foods, such as butter, cream, and fatty meats, can also contribute to weight gain and increase the risk of heart disease and stroke. Foods high in sugar, such as glucose, fructose, and corn syrup, can also lead to weight gain and obesity.

Physical Inactivity: A lack of physical activity can also contribute to weight gain and obesity. Sitting for long periods of time, such as at work or in front of a screen, can lead to weight gain and poor overall health. It is important to engage in regular physical activity, such as walking, cycling, or going to the gym, to maintain a healthy weight.Other factors, such as genetics, medications, and sleep patterns, can also contribute to weight.

3. WHY SHOULD WE LOSE EXTRA WEIGHT?

Maintaining a healthy weight is essential for good health and overall wellbeing. Extra weight can cause a range of health problems, such as increased risk of heart disease, diabetes, and other chronic diseases. It can also lead to a decrease in energy levels, as well as mental and physical fatigue. Therefore, losing extra weight can help you to reduce your risk of developing these conditions, as well as improving your overall health and quality of life.

There are many benefits to losing extra weight, apart from reducing the risk of health problems. The most obvious ones are the improved physical appearance, increased confidence, and improved physical fitness. Losing weight can also lead to improved mental health, as feelings of self-esteem and self-worth can increase.

Losing weight is not an easy task, but it is possible with the right approach. The key is to combine a healthy diet and regular physical activity. A healthy diet should include plenty of fruits, vegetables, whole grains, and lean proteins, as well as reducing processed and junk foods.
Regular physical activity is important to keep your metabolism going and to burn off excess calories. It can be anything from walking, running, or cycling to taking up a sport or joining an exercise class.

In addition to diet and exercise, there are other strategies you can use to help you lose extra weight. Setting realistic goals, tracking your progress, and replacing bad habits with good ones, such as cutting back on sugar and processed foods, can all help. Also, consider stress-reduction techniques like yoga and meditation, as stress can be a trigger for weight gain. Finally, don't forget to get enough sleep, as this can affect your energy levels and make it harder to reach your weight-loss goals.

Losing extra weight can have many benefits, both physical and psychological. By combining a healthy diet, regular physical activity, and other helpful strategies, you can reach your weight-loss goals and improve your overall health and wellbeing.

3.1. Benefits of Losing Weight

Losing excess weight is one of the most important things you can do for your health. Not only can it help you look and feel better, but it can also have far-reaching benefits on your physical and emotional wellbeing. Here are some of the most significant benefits of losing weight.

Improved Physical Health: The most obvious benefit of losing weight is improved physical health. Carrying around extra weight is associated with an increased risk of a number of health concerns, including type 2 diabetes, heart disease, stroke, and even some types of cancer. Losing weight can reduce your risk of many of these conditions.

In addition, shedding excess weight can help ease joint pain, improve your breathing and cardiovascular endurance, and increase your energy levels. People who lose weight may also find that their blood pressure and cholesterol levels improve.

Improved Mental Health: In addition to physical health benefits, losing weight can also have a positive impact on your mental health. Research suggests that people who are overweight or obese are more likely to suffer from depression and anxiety. Losing weight can improve self-confidence, body image, and overall wellbeing.

Research also indicates that people who lose weight tend to get more quality sleep. Quality sleep is important for mental and physical health, and it can help to reduce stress. Plus, getting more sleep can make it easier to stick to a healthier lifestyle overall. Being overweight or obese can increase the risk of sleep apnea, a condition where a person's breathing is briefly interrupted during sleep. Losing weight can help improve sleep quality.

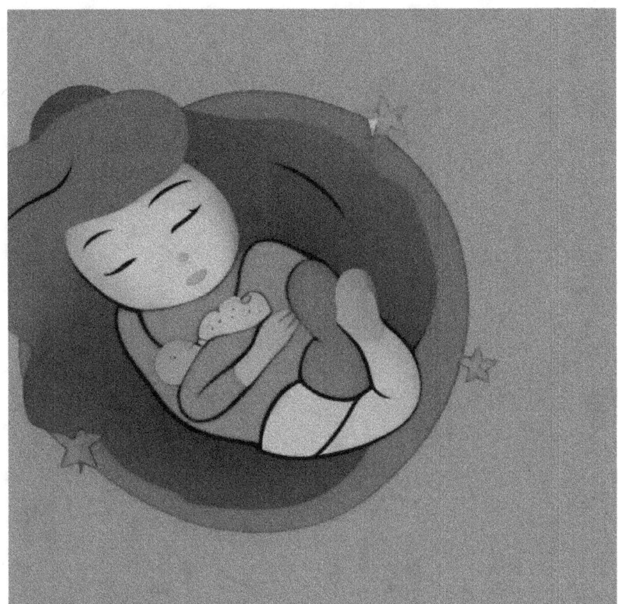

Increased Mobility: Carrying extra weight can make it harder to move around, and it can even limit your mobility. Losing weight can help you to move more freely and with less effort. It can also help you to do more physical activities that you may have found difficult before. Plus, increased mobility can help to reduce the risk of falls and other injuries. Carrying extra weight can make it more difficult to move around and be active. Losing weight can help increase energy levels and make it easier to engage in physical activity.

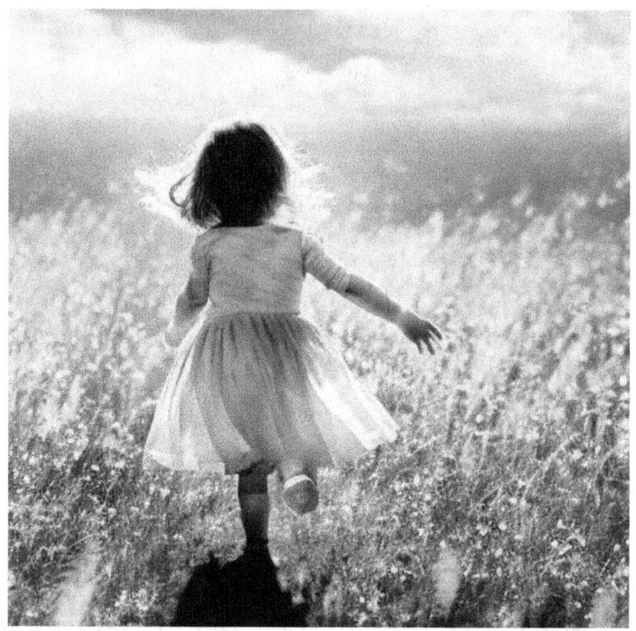

Improved Quality of Life: Finally, losing weight can lead to improved quality of life. Research suggests that people who lose weight experience improved physical and mental functioning and report greater satisfaction with their lives. They are also more likely to engage in activities that are important for overall wellbeing, such as exercising, socializing, and participating in leisure activities.

Health benefits: Being overweight or obese can increase the risk of a number of health conditions, such as heart disease, diabetes, and certain cancers. Losing weight can help reduce the risk of these conditions and improve overall health.

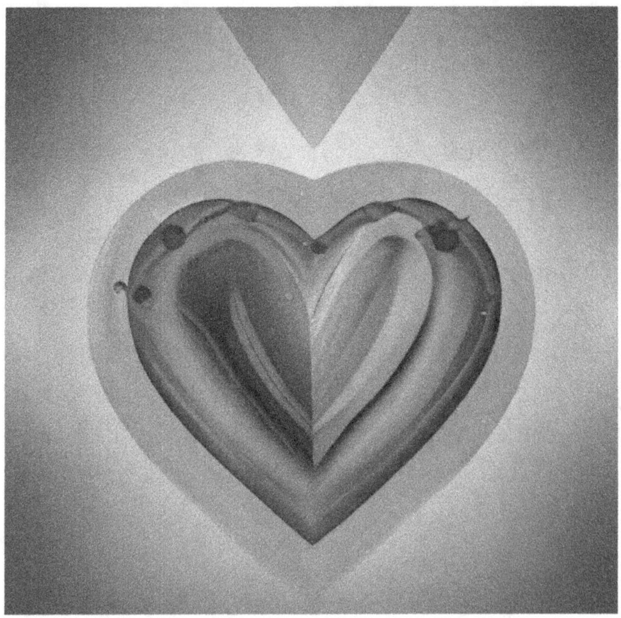

Improving self-esteem and confidence: Many people feel self-conscious about their weight and may feel more confident and positive about themselves when they lose weight.

Improving athletic performance: Extra weight can make it more difficult to perform in sports or other physical activities. Losing weight can help improve performance in these areas.

It's important to note that weight loss should be done in a healthy and sustainable way, and not based on fad diets or extreme measures that can harm your health.
Additionally, weight loss should not be the only goal, rather overall health and well-being. It's important to talk to your doctor or a registered dietitian before starting any weight loss program, especially if you have any health conditions.

Overall, the benefits of losing weight are far-reaching and can have a dramatic impact on your physical and emotional wellbeing. It is important to talk to your doctor before beginning any kind of weight loss plan, so that you can create an individualized plan that is tailored.

Do you feel like you're stuck in an endless cycle of failed diets and workout regimens? Do you want to shed the excess weight, but don't know how to get started? Have faith - you can do it! With the right motivation and focus, you can reach your weight loss goals.

When it comes to motivation, it's important to remember that there's no one size fits all approach. Everyone is motivated differently, so it's important to find what works best for you. Here are some tips to help you get motivated to lose weight through diet and exercise.

3.2. Find Your Why

The first step to finding motivation is to determine why you want to lose weight. What's the reason behind it? Do you want to reduce your risk of chronic disease? Do you want to feel more confident in your body? Do you want to increase your energy levels?

Take some time to think about why you want to lose weight. Write down your reasons and keep them somewhere visible, like your fridge or bathroom mirror. This will serve as a constant reminder of why you're embarking on this journey.

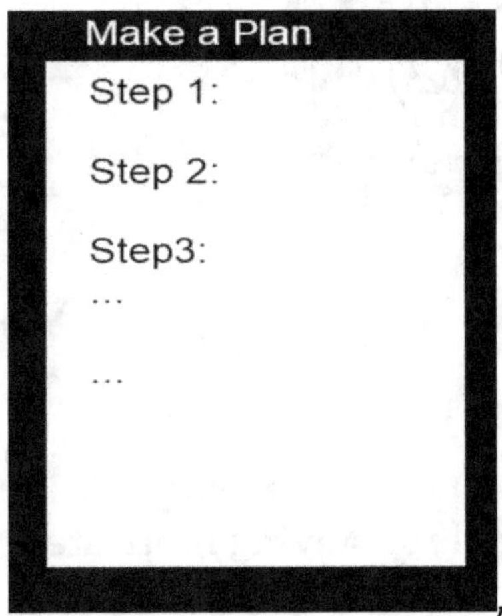

Make a Plan:

Now that you know why you want to lose weight, it's time to set a plan. Start by deciding what type of diet you want to follow and look for exercise routines that you enjoy. Talk to your doctor to make sure that it's safe for you to start a diet and exercise routine. Once you have a plan in place, write down your goals – both short-term and long-term. These goals should be realistic and attainable. Break them down into small steps that you can take each day. This will make the goals easier to achieve, and help keep you motivated.

Find A Support System:

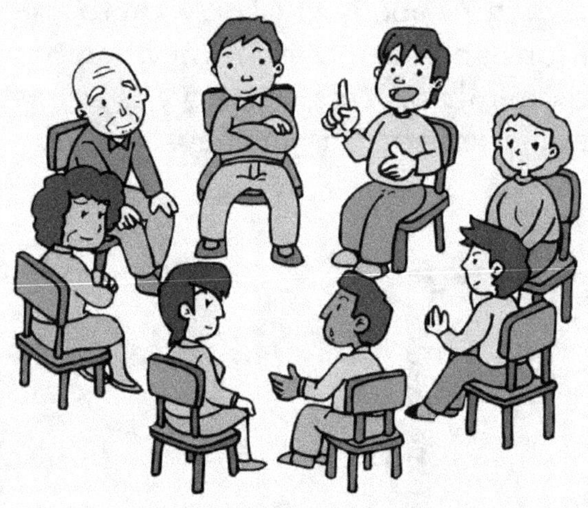

Having a good support system is essential for staying motivated. A support system can provide encouragement and accountability. If you can't find someone in person, look for online communities or forums. There are lots of different weight loss communities out there, so you can find one that fits your needs.

It can also help to follow weight loss stories on social media. Seeing real people's successes can inspire you to keep going.

In conclusion, this chapter has provided an overview of the importance of planning in weight loss and the steps involved in creating a successful weight loss plan. We discussed the problems associated with being overweight, including the health risks and the impact on overall quality of life. We also highlighted the many benefits of losing weight, including improved physical health, increased energy, and improved self-esteem.

"As we move on to the next chapter, we will delve deeper into the importance of both proper nutrition and exercise when it comes to achieving weight loss goals. In this chapter, we will discuss the different types of foods that can help support weight loss efforts and provide tips for creating a balanced and nutritious meal plan. We will also explore various exercise options and the role they play in burning calories and building muscle."

4. PLANNING

Weight loss can be a daunting task, but it doesn't have to be. There are simple steps you can take to jumpstart your journey to a healthier you. When it comes to weight loss, it's important to set realistic goals. Don't be too hard on yourself or set goals too high. Instead, focus on smaller, achievable goals that you can reach and celebrate. This will help keep you motivated, while also avoiding disappointment and frustration.

Tracking your progress is an essential part of any successful weight loss journey. Keep track of the foods you eat, your exercise routine, and your weight. This will help you stay on track and keep motivated as you continue on your journey. Rather than cutting out all unhealthy foods, find healthier alternatives instead. Many unhealthy snacks can be replaced with healthy options like fruits, vegetables, and nuts. If you're trying to cut down on eating takeout, try making healthy meals at home using fresh ingredients.

Exercise is a great way to stay in shape and lose weight. Start by adding a few simple activities to your daily routine such as walking or jogging. As you get more comfortable, begin to incorporate more intense workouts such as weight training or HIIT. Having a support system is an important part of any weight loss journey. If you know someone who is also trying to lose weight, join forces and encourage each other to stay on track. If you don't have someone in your circle that you can rely on, there are plenty of online communities and forums that offer support.

Weight loss doesn't have to be a daunting task. By following these simple steps and staying motivated, you can jumpstart your journey to a healthier you.

4.1. Plan your weight lose Journey

Weight loss can be a challenging journey, but planning and preparation are key to success. In this chapter, we will discuss the importance of planning in weight loss and provide an overview of the steps involved in creating a successful weight loss plan.

Setting Realistic Goals

The first step in planning a weight loss journey is to set realistic goals. It is important to determine a healthy weight range for your body type, taking into account factors such as muscle mass, height, and age. Setting achievable and measurable goals, both short-term and long-term, can help you stay motivated and on track. For example, setting a goal to lose 1-2 pounds per week, or to reach a certain weight within a certain timeframe, can help you stay focused on your progress.

Assessing Your Current Lifestyle

To effectively plan your weight loss journey, it's important to take an honest look at your current eating and exercise habits. Understanding the role of stress, sleep, and other factors in weight loss can also help you identify areas that need improvement. Once you have a clear picture of your current lifestyle, you can make a plan to address any areas of concern. This might include setting a regular sleep schedule, reducing stress through mindfulness practices, or incorporating more physical activity into your day.

Creating A Weight Loss Plan

Once you have assessed your current lifestyle and set realistic goals, you can begin to create a weight loss plan. Choosing a diet that works for you is a key element of this plan. Low-carb, low-fat, and other dietary approaches can all be effective, but it's important to find one that fits your individual needs and preferences. Developing an exercise routine that fits your schedule and fitness level is also important, whether that means taking a daily walk, joining a gym, or signing up for a fitness class.

Incorporating Behavior Change Strategies

Incorporating behavior change strategies can help you make lasting changes to your eating and exercise habits. Some effective strategies include keeping a food diary, setting reminders to move throughout the day, or finding a workout buddy to help keep you accountable. Building a support system of friends and family, or joining a weight loss support group, can also be helpful.

Staying On Track And Overcoming Obstacles

Even with the best of plans, obstacles can arise that make it difficult to stay on track. The key is to stay motivated and find ways to overcome these obstacles. Keeping a positive attitude, reminding yourself of your goals, and finding healthy ways to cope with stress can help you stay on track. It's also important to be flexible and adjust your plan as needed. If you slip up and have a bad day, don't give up. Instead, refocus and get back on track.

Weight loss is a journey that requires planning and commitment. By setting realistic goals, assessing your current lifestyle, creating a weight loss plan, incorporating behavior change strategies, and staying motivated, you can increase your chances of success. Remember to be kind to yourself, weight loss is not easy and it's not a linear process, it's okay to have setbacks, but don't let them discourage you. With determination and persistence, you can reach your weight loss goals and improve your overall health and well-being.

4.2. Do you want to motivate someone else to lose weight?

Motivating someone to lose weight can be a challenging task, as weight loss is a personal and complex process that can be affected by many factors, such as genetics, lifestyle, and psychological well-being. However, there are some strategies that can help to motivate people to lose weight:

Be supportive: Encourage and support the person in their weight loss journey, listen to their concerns and offer help when needed.

Provide education: Share reliable information about weight loss, nutrition, and exercise to help the person make informed decisions.

Set realistic goals: Help the person set realistic and achievable weight loss goals, and provide them with a plan to reach those goals.

Create a positive environment: Create an environment that supports healthy habits, such as stocking the pantry with healthy food options, and encouraging regular physical activity.
Use positive reinforcement: Recognize and acknowledge the person's progress and accomplishments, and celebrate their successes.
Be a good role model: Lead by example, and make healthy choices yourself, people will be more motivated to lose weight if they see others doing it successfully.

Encourage self-compassion: Help the person develop a more positive relationship with their body, and encourage them to be kind and compassionate with themselves throughout the process.

It's important to remember that weight loss is a personal journey, and each person's motivation will be unique to them. Be patient, kind and understanding and help the person to identify the reason why they want to lose weight, and help them to focus on the benefits of a healthy lifestyle.

Chapter Summary/Key Takeaways:

In conclusion, we began by setting realistic goals and assessing your current lifestyle to identify areas that need improvement. From there, we discussed creating a weight loss plan that fits your individual needs and preferences, and incorporating behavior change strategies to support your weight loss efforts. We also covered strategies for staying on track and overcoming obstacles that may arise during your journey. It is important to remember that weight loss is a journey and it's not always easy. It requires commitment, determination, and persistence.

However, with the right plan and the right mindset, you can achieve your weight loss goals and improve your overall health and well-being. Remember to always consult your healthcare provider before starting any weight loss journey and be kind to yourself, weight loss is not a one-time event, it's a lifelong journey.

Losing weight can be a challenging process, but with a well-thought-out plan and the right mindset, it is possible to achieve your weight loss goals. Here are some steps to help you plan to lose weight:

Set realistic goals: Determine how much weight you want to lose and set a specific, measurable and achievable goal.

Create a calorie deficit: To lose weight, you need to burn more calories than you consume. Keep track of the calories you consume and burn through exercise, and make sure you are in a calorie deficit.

Incorporate regular physical activity: Exercise is an important component of weight loss, as it helps to burn calories and build muscle. Aim for at least 30 minutes of moderate-intensity exercise most days of the week.

Make healthy food choices: Eating a balanced diet that is high in fruits, vegetables, lean proteins, and whole grains will help to keep you full and satisfied while providing your body with the nutrients it needs.

Be consistent: Losing weight takes time and effort, so it's important to stick with your plan even when progress seems slow or when you encounter obstacles.
Keep track of progress: Keep track of your weight and measurements, and take progress photos to help you stay motivated.

Get support: Surround yourself with people who will support and encourage you, consider joining a weight loss support group or working with a dietitian or personal trainer.

Be flexible: Life happens, and plans change, be willing to adapt your plan as needed, and remember that setbacks are not failures, they are opportunities to learn and grow.
Remember that weight loss is not a one-size-fits-all process, so it's important to consult with your doctor or a registered dietitian to find a plan that works for you, and it is also important to be patient and persistent in your efforts.

"As we move on to the next chapter, we will delve deeper into the importance of both proper nutrition and exercise when it comes to achieving weight loss goals. In this chapter, we will discuss the different types of foods that can help support weight loss efforts and provide tips for creating a balanced and nutritious meal plan.

We will also explore various exercise options and the role they play in burning calories and building muscle."

5. FOOD AND EXERCISES

When it comes to healthy weight loss, what you eat is just as important as how much you eat. Eating the right foods can help your body burn fat and build muscle, while providing you with the energy you need to stay active and healthy. To achieve your weight loss goals, it's important to incorporate a variety of foods into your diet. Fruits and vegetables are essential to any balanced diet. They are high in essential vitamins and minerals, but low in calories.

Eating a variety of fruits and vegetables can also help you get all of the important vitamins and minerals your body needs. For example, adding an apple to your breakfast could help you get extra Vitamin C and dietary fiber. Eating dark, leafy greens is a great way to get your daily vitamins and minerals. Whole grains are another important component of any healthy diet. Eating whole grains can help you stay fuller for longer and help your body absorb essential vitamins and minerals. Quinoa, oats, and brown rice are all healthy whole grains that you can easily incorporate into your meals.

In addition to fruits and vegetables, lean proteins can help you with your weight loss goals. Lean proteins, such as chicken, fish, and eggs, are low in fat and calories, and high in essential amino acids. They can and brown rice are all healthy whole grains that you can easily incorporate into your meals.

In addition to fruits and vegetables, lean proteins can help you with your weight loss goals. Lean proteins, such as chicken, fish, and eggs, are low in fat and calories, and high in essential amino acids. They can help keep you full and aid in muscle growth. Lean proteins can also help your body burn fat faster.

Fat can be a tricky component of any diet. While some fats are essential for healthy living, it's important to get the right kinds of fat. Healthy fats, like those found in nuts, avocados, and olive oil, are a great way to get essential nutrients while still keeping your calorie intake low.

Finally, healthy drinks can help you with your weight loss goals. Drinking plenty of water is essential for staying hydrated and flushing out toxins. Low-calorie, unsweetened drinks like tea are a great way to get your fluids without extra calories.

Eating the right kinds of food can help you achieve your weight loss goals. Incorporating a variety of fruits and vegetables, whole grains, lean proteins, and healthy fats.

Carbohydrates, proteins, and vitamins are all essential macronutrients that our bodies need to function properly. Each of these nutrients plays an important role in maintaining our health and well-being. In this chapter, we will explore what types of foods contain these nutrients, how much we need, and how to include them in our diets.

Carbohydrates:

Carbohydrates are a type of macronutrient that our bodies use as a primary source of energy. They are found in a wide variety of foods, including fruits, vegetables, grains, and legumes. Some examples of foods that are high in carbohydrates include potatoes, rice, pasta, bread, and cereal.

The recommended daily intake of carbohydrates varies depending on your age, sex, and activity level. However, most adults should aim to consume between 130 and 225 grams of carbohydrates per day.

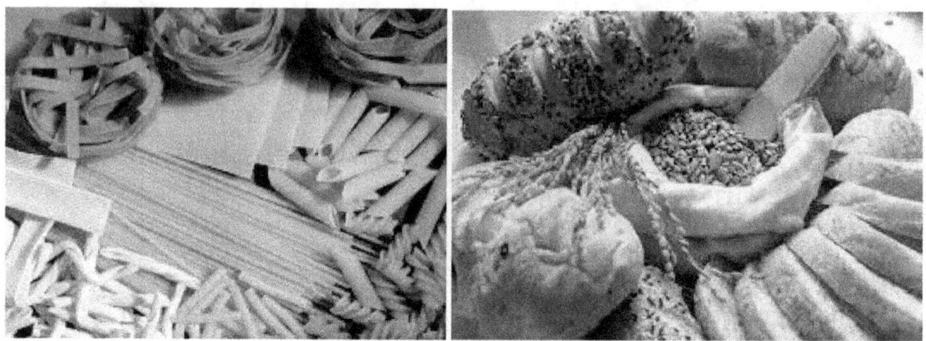

Proteins:

Proteins are essential macronutrients that our bodies use to build and repair tissues. They are found in a variety of foods, including meats, dairy products, eggs, and plant-based sources such as beans and lentils. Some examples of foods that are high in protein include chicken, fish, beef, and Greek yogurt. The recommended daily intake of protein varies depending on your age, sex, and activity level. However, most adults should aim to consume between 46 and 56 grams of protein per day.

Proteins are essential macronutrients that our bodies use to build and repair tissues. They are found in a variety of foods, including meats, dairy products, eggs, and plant-based sources such as beans and lentils.

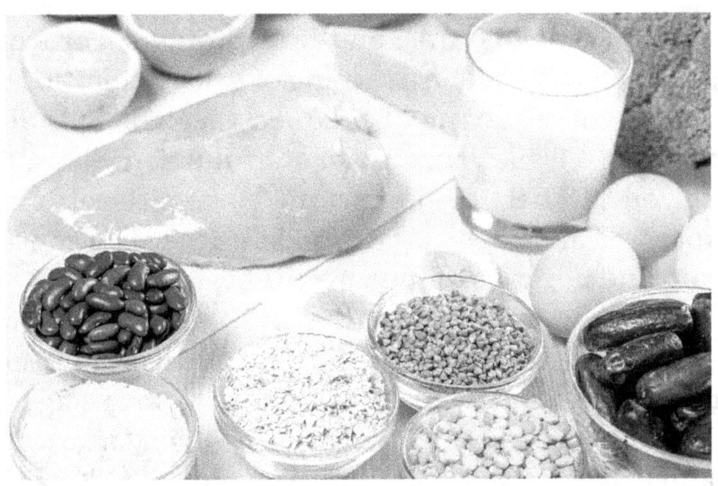

Some examples of foods that are high in protein include chicken, fish, beef, and Greek yogurt.

The recommended daily intake of protein varies depending on your age, sex, and activity level. However, most adults should aim to consume between 46 and 56 grams of protein per day.

Vitamins:

Vitamins are essential micronutrients that our bodies need to function properly. They are found in a variety of foods, including fruits, vegetables, and fortified foods. Some examples of foods that are high in vitamins include oranges, spinach, and fortified cereal.

The recommended daily intake of vitamins varies depending on your age, sex, and activity level. However, most adults should aim to consume a variety of vitamins daily, including vitamin A, vitamin C, vitamin D, and vitamin E.

To include these essential macronutrients in your diet, it is important to have a well-balanced and varied diet. A good way to start is to make sure you are consuming a variety of fruits and vegetables, whole grains, and lean proteins. For example, a balanced meal could include a serving of grilled chicken, a serving of brown rice, and a serving of steamed vegetables. Additionally, it is important to limit your intake of of nutrient-dense foods in your diet, you can help to support your overall health and well-being. Processed and high-calorie foods, as they can contribute to weight gain and negatively impact your health.

It is also important to consult with a healthcare professional or a registered dietitian to determine the specific macronutrient needs for your body based on your current health status, age, sex and level of physical activity. They can also help you to develop a healthy and balanced meal plan to meet your specific needs.

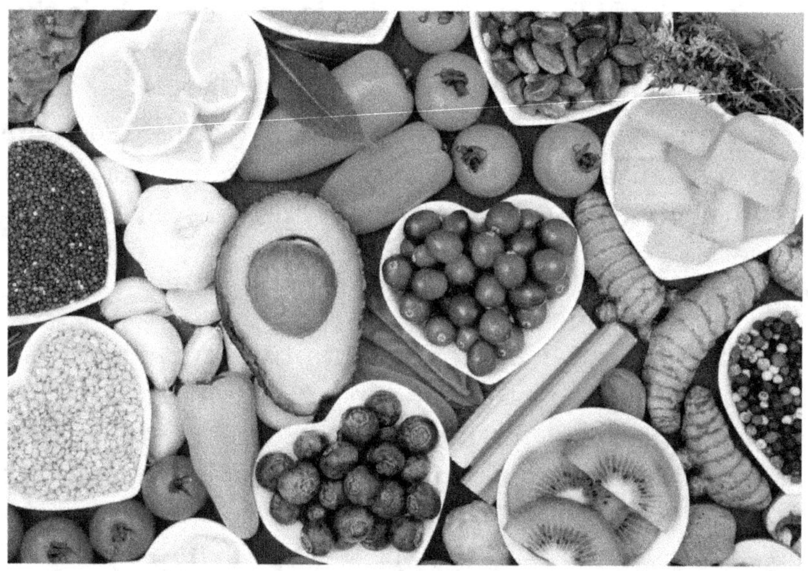

In conclusion, carbohydrates, proteins and vitamins are essential macronutrients that our bodies need to function properly. To maintain a healthy and balanced diet, it is important to consume a variety of foods that contain these nutrients, including fruits, vegetables, and whole grains. By including a variety of nutrient-dense foods in your diet, you can help to support your overall health and well-being.

6. PLAN YOUR DIET

There are many foods that can be helpful for weight loss, as they are nutrient-dense and can help you feel full and satisfied while also providing your body with the necessary nutrients. Some examples include:

Fruits and vegetables: These foods are low in calories and high in fiber, vitamins, and minerals. They can help you feel full and satisfied, and are also beneficial for overall health.

Whole grains: Whole grains such as oats, quinoa, brown rice, and whole wheat bread are high in fiber and can help you feel full and satisfied. They also provide your body with important nutrients such as B vitamins, iron, and zinc.

Lean protein: Foods such as chicken, fish, tofu, and legumes are high in protein and can help you feel full and satisfied. Protein also helps to preserve muscle mass while you are losing weight.

Nuts and seeds: They are rich in healthy fats, protein, and fiber and can help you feel full and satisfied. They are also high in nutrients such as magnesium, potassium, and zinc.

Healthy fats: Foods such as avocado, olive oil, and nuts are high in healthy fats and can help you feel full and satisfied. They also provide important nutrients such as vitamin E, potassium, and magnesium.

Water: Drinking water can help you feel full, and it has zero calories. Drinking water before meals can also help you eat less.

It's also important to note that weight loss is not only about the foods that you eat, but also about the quantity of food, and the balance of macronutrients (carbohydrates, proteins and fats) you consume. A balance diet and moderate portion size is the key to losing weight. Additionally, it's important to talk to your doctor or a registered dietitian before making any major changes to your diet, especially if you have any health conditions.

6.1. Popular Diet Plans to Lose Weight

For those looking to shed a few pounds, there are countless diet plans available to help you reach your goal. No matter your lifestyle, there are many options that can fit into your life and help you to lose weight and maintain a healthy lifestyle. Here are some popular diet plans that may be suitable for you.

The Mediterranean Diet:

The Mediterranean Diet is a way of eating based on the traditional food patterns of the countries surrounding the Mediterranean Sea. It is widely considered one of the healthiest diets in the world and is associated with many health benefits, including weight loss and a reduced risk of chronic diseases such as heart disease, type 2 diabetes, and certain cancers.

The Mediterranean Diet is rich in whole, unprocessed foods, including:

Fruits and vegetables: These are the cornerstone of the Mediterranean Diet and should make up a large part of daily meals.

Whole grains: Whole grain breads, pastas, and cereals should replace refined grains.
Nuts and seeds: These are high in healthy fats, fiber, and protein, making them a great snack or addition to meals.
Legumes: Beans, lentils, and chickpeas are good sources of protein and fiber, and should be incorporated regularly.

Fish and seafood: Fish, especially fatty fish such as salmon, should be eaten at least two times per week.

Olive oil: This is the primary source of healthy fat in the Mediterranean Diet, and should be used in place of unhealthy fats like butter.

The Mediterranean Diet also includes moderate amounts of dairy products, eggs, and poultry, and small amounts of red meat. It emphasizes the use of herbs and spices to flavor food, instead of salt and sugar. Wine is consumed in moderation with meals.

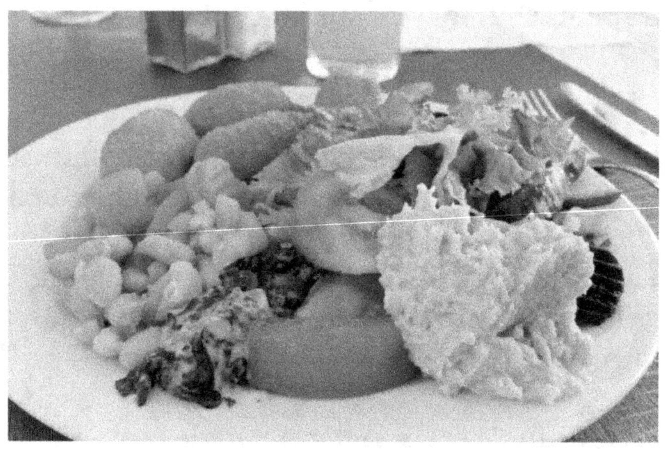

In conclusion, the Mediterranean Diet is a healthy, balanced way of eating that has been shown to have many health benefits, including weight loss and a reduced risk of chronic diseases. Incorporating whole, unprocessed foods and limiting processed foods, sugar, and unhealthy fats is the key to following the Mediterranean Diet and achieving good health.

The DASH Diet:

The DASH Diet is a popular and highly recommended way of eating for overall health and wellness. The acronym stands for "Dietary Approaches to Stop Hypertension", and it was designed for the purpose of lowering blood pressure. The DASH diet emphasizes eating whole foods in their natural state, such as fresh fruits and vegetables, whole grains, and lean proteins. It also recommends limiting processed foods, added sugars, and salt, as well as consuming fewer saturated and trans fats.

The DASH diet is rich in many essential nutrients such as potassium, magnesium, and calcium, which help to lower blood pressure by promoting healthy blood vessel functioning. Additionally, the DASH diet encourages consuming certain 'superfoods' such as leafy greens, walnuts, and avocados, which are known to be particularly nutrient-dense. Eating regular meals and snacks, instead of skipping meals, can also help to maintain healthy blood pressure levels.

The DASH diet also promotes physical activity, which is an important part of a healthy lifestyle. Regular exercise can help to reduce stress levels, improve mood, and promote heart health. Additionally, it can help to regulate blood sugar levels, which is often an issue for those with hypertension.

In general, the DASH diet is a great option for those looking to maintain healthy blood pressure levels. It is a balanced and nutritious way of eating that emphasizes consuming unprocessed, whole foods and limiting added sugars, salt, and unhealthy fats. With regular physical activity and a balanced diet, it is possible to lower blood pressure and improve overall health.

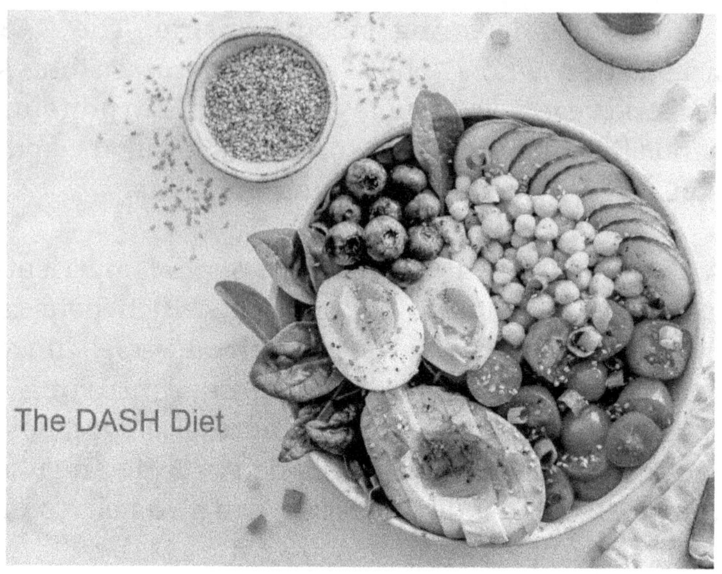

Intermittent Fasting:

Intermittent fasting is a popular diet trend that has been taking the health and wellness industry by storm. Intermittent fasting involves alternating between periods of eating and periods of abstaining from food. This type of fasting is becoming increasingly popular due to the potential health benefits it offers. Studies have shown that intermittent fasting can help reduce weight, improve cardiovascular health, reduce inflammation, and improve mental clarity.

Intermittent fasting typically involves periods of fasting ranging from 12-36 hours. During this time, no food is consumed, but water, tea, coffee and other non-caloric beverages are allowed. During the eating period, people are allowed to eat whatever they choose, but it is important to make sure to get enough nutrients and maintain a balanced diet.

Intermittent fasting has been shown to increase metabolic

flexibility, which means the body can easily switch between burning glucose and fat for energy. This can help reduce weight and optimize metabolic health. Intermittent fasting also helps reduce inflammation, which can be beneficial for people with chronic diseases. Additionally, research has shown that intermittent fasting can help improve cognition and mental clarity.

Intermittent fasting is not an easy diet, and may not be suitable for everyone. It is important to speak with your doctor before starting any new diet or health regimen. Intermittent fasting should not be done in place of regular meals, but rather as a supplement to a balanced diet. It is also important to make sure to get enough vitamins and minerals during the eating periods.

Intermittent fasting can be an effective tool for anyone looking to maximize their health. It can help reduce weight, improve metabolic health, reduce inflammation, and increase mental clarity. It is important to speak with your doctor before starting intermittent fasting to make sure it is a safe and appropriate option for you. With proper guidance, intermittent fasting can be an effective way to reach your health and wellness goals.

The Atkins Diet:

The Atkins Diet, also known as the Atkins Nutritional Approach, is a low-carbohydrate diet that has become popular over the past few decades for its purported weight-loss benefits. It is based on the concept of reducing carbohydrate intake in order to induce a state of ketosis, which is when the body starts burning fat for energy instead of glucose. The diet consists of several phases, each of which encourages a different level of carbohydrate intake and is designed to help adherents reach their desired weight-loss goals.

The first phase is the Induction phase, which is the most

restrictive as it limits carbohydrate intake to less than 20 grams per day. This low-carbohydrate intake helps to kick-start the process of ketosis, and typically lasts for two weeks or until the desired weight-loss target is reached. After this phase, adherents gradually increase their carbohydrate intake in increments of 5-10 grams per day, until the desired level of carbohydrate intake is reached.

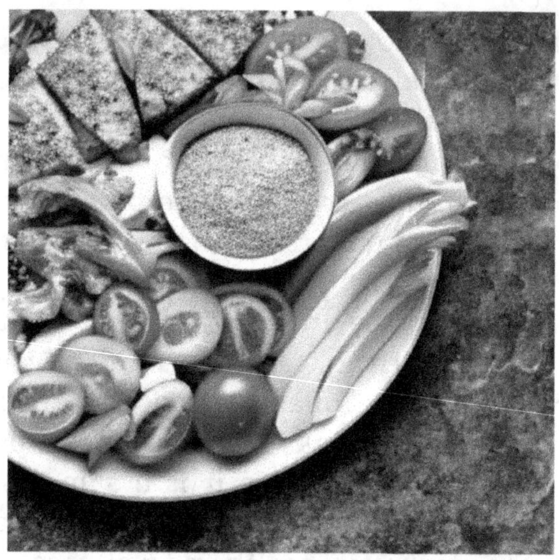

The Atkins Diet also encourages its followers to eat lean proteins, good fats, and fresh fruits and vegetables. These nutrient-dense foods provide the body with the necessary energy to maintain a healthy lifestyle. Additionally, moderate-intensity exercises are encouraged to help enhance the results.

In conclusion, the Atkins Diet is an effective and safe way to lose weight. It helps to kick-start ketosis, and encourages its followers to maintain a healthy lifestyle by eating nutrient-dense foods and engaging in moderate-intensity exercises. While the diet does have its critics, it has nonetheless become a popular choice for those looking to lose weight.

The Paleo Diet:

The Paleo Diet is a dietary plan that focuses on eating the same types of foods that were eaten by humans during the Paleolithic era. It is a low-carb diet that avoids processed foods, grains, and dairy. Instead, followers of the Paleo Diet focus on consuming foods like fruits, vegetables, nuts, seeds, and lean proteins such as fish and poultry.

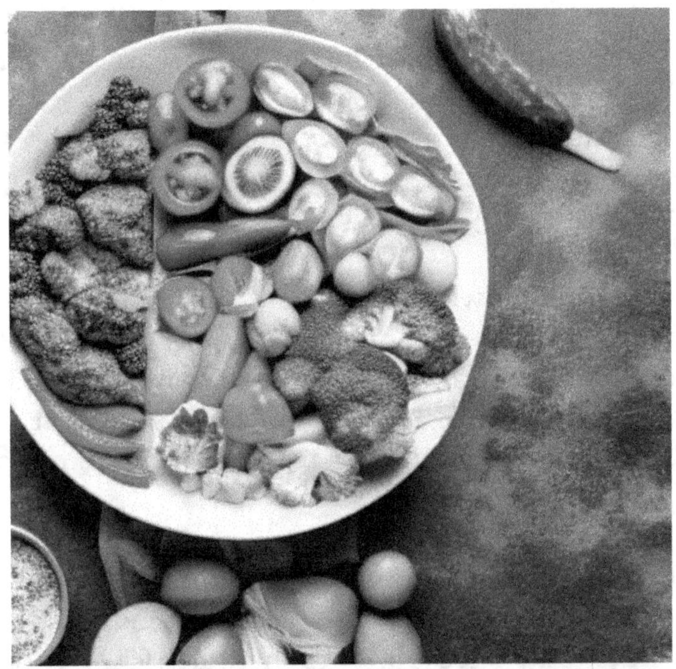

This diet is often used for weight loss as it helps to reduce calories by eliminating processed and sugary foods. Additionally, Paleo followers find that eating nutrient-dense foods helps them to feel more satiated and that naturally occurring fats help to keep them feeling fuller for longer. Finally, this diet also avoids many common food allergens, which can help to reduce inflammation. All of these aspects can help to support healthy and sustainable weight loss.

For many people, the goal of a healthier lifestyle includes reducing body weight. Losing weight can help improve physical fitness, reduce the risk of certain health conditions, and boost overall confidence. However, dieting can be a complicated process and require careful consideration. Here, we will discuss three common diet plans to reduce weight, including the ketogenic diet, low-carb diet, and intermittent fasting.

The Ketogenic Diet:

Ketogenic diets are very popular these days as they are linked to weight loss, risk reduction of metabolic diseases, and improved cognitive performance. A ketogenic diet is a low-carbohydrate and high-fat diet, where the body breaks down stored fat into molecules called ketones, which are then used for energy instead of glucose from carbohydrates.

When a person follows a ketogenic diet, the body enters a metabolic state called ketosis. This means that the body is burning fat for energy instead of glucose from carbohydrates. Ketosis can provide numerous health benefits, including a boost in energy, improved cognitive performance, better blood sugar control, and increased weight loss.

When following a ketogenic diet, it is important to choose healthy sources of fat and protein. These include foods like fatty fish, avocados, nuts, and olive oil. Carbohydrates should be limited, focusing on small amounts of vegetables, fruit, and whole grains. Eating adequate amounts of healthy fat is important to provide energy and to help the body enter ketosis.

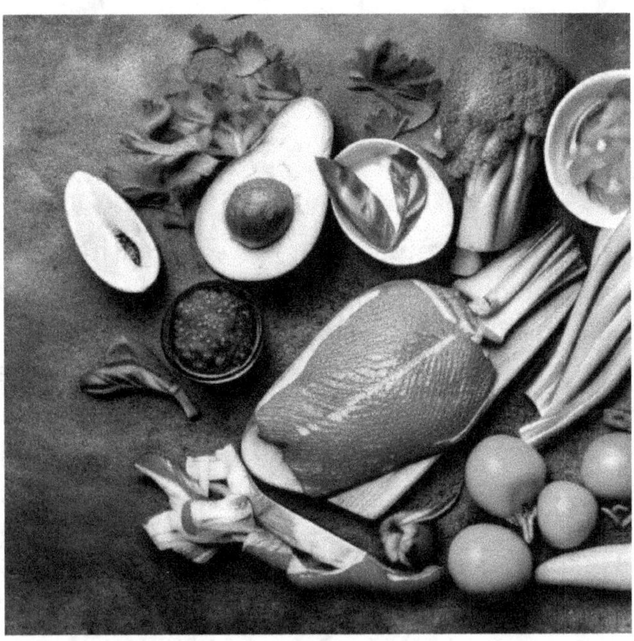

Eating too much protein can cause the body to produce glucose, which can take the body out of ketosis. It is important to track macronutrient intake to make sure that the body is in ketosis. Tracking ketone levels can help to ensure the body is producing enough ketones.

In addition to following a healthy ketogenic diet, hydration is important for maintaining ketosis. Drinking plenty of water can help to manage sugar cravings and improve energy levels. Supplementation with minerals and electrolytes can help to maintain electrolyte balance, as well as to help the body reach and remain in ketosis.

Overall, ketogenic diets are a great way to lose weight, reduce risk of metabolic diseases, and improve cognitive performance. Eating healthy sources of fat and protein, limiting carbohydrate intake, and tracking macronutrient intake are all important for maintaining ketosis and the associated health benefits. Additionally, staying hydrated and supplementing with minerals and electrolytes can help to ensure the body stays in a healthy, ketogenic state.

Low-Carb Diet:

A low-carb diet is a popular way of eating that eliminates or greatly reduces carbohydrate intake from one's diet. By limiting carbohydrates, the body is forced to burn fat for fuel instead of carbohydrates. This is known as ketosis, and it has been shown to increase weight loss and reduce the risk of developing certain chronic diseases. A low-carb diet typically restricts the intake of grains, fruits, and starchy vegetables while increasing the amount of proteins, fats, and vegetables consumed.

There are many benefits to taking on a low-carb diet. Studies have shown that limiting carbohydrate intake can help with weight loss and improve metabolic health. Additionally, a low-carb diet can help to reduce risk factors for diabetes, heart disease, and some types of cancer. It can also help to reduce symptoms of some neurological disorders, such as Alzheimer's disease, and improve overall mental health.

When following a low-carb diet, it is important to focus on nutrient-dense, high-quality foods. Processed foods, added sugars, and unhealthy fats should be avoided as much as possible. Instead, focus on eating lean proteins, healthy fats, and non-starchy vegetables. Healthy fats are especially important as they provide the energy needed to fuel the body and brain. Good sources include avocados, nuts, nut butters, and olive oil.

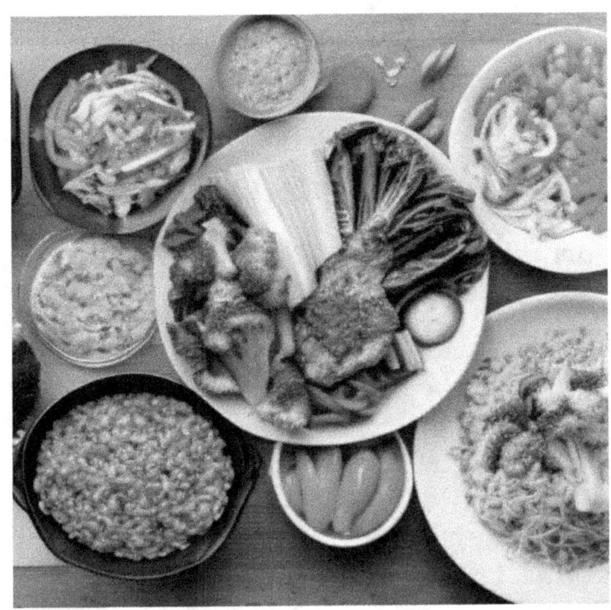

In addition to eating healthy fats and proteins, it is important to drink plenty of water and other non-caloric beverages. This will help to keep the body hydrated and can help to reduce cravings for sweets and other unhealthy foods. Additionally, if possible, try to get enough sleep and exercise regularly. These lifestyle changes can help to support a healthy metabolism and overall well-being.

Overall, a low-carb diet can be a great way to support weight loss goals and improve metabolic health. It is important to make sure to focus on nutrient-dense foods and follow a healthy lifestyle while on the diet. With the right plan and a bit of dedication, a low-carb diet can be an effective way to achieve health and wellness goals.

6.2. Some frequently asked questions

➤ **Is just drinking milk for dinner time is fine for a month?**

Drinking milk as your sole source of nutrition at dinnertime for a month is not a balanced or healthy diet plan. Milk is a good source of calcium and other nutrients, but it does not provide enough essential vitamins and minerals to sustain a healthy diet. A balanced diet should include a variety of different food groups, including fruits, vegetables, whole grains, lean protein, and healthy fats. Additionally, it is important to consider food allergies, intolerance and other medical conditions when planning a diet. It is always best to consult a healthcare professional or a registered dietitian before making any significant changes to your diet.

➤ **Is just drinking milk at dinner reduce weight?**

Drinking milk at dinner, or any other meal, will not reduce weight in and of itself. In fact, consuming too many calories, whether they come from milk or other foods, can contribute to weight gain. To lose weight, it is important to create a calorie deficit by burning more calories than you consume. This can be achieved by reducing calorie intake, increasing physical activity, or a combination of both.

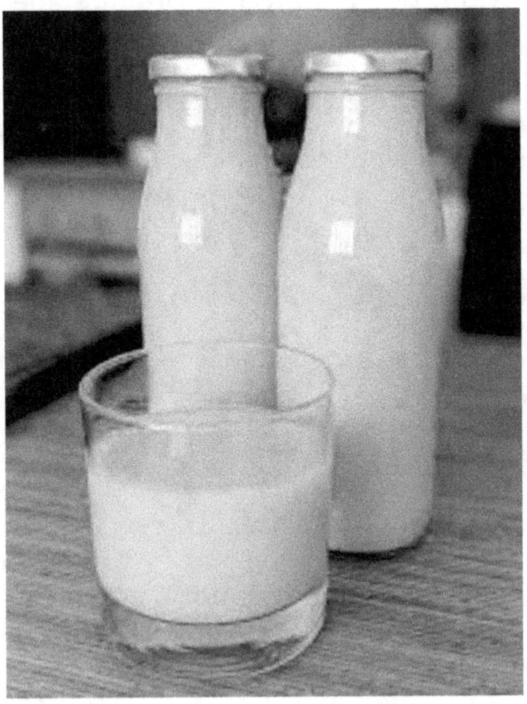

Milk can be part of a weight-loss diet as long as it is consumed in moderation and part of a balanced diet. Milk provides some important nutrients like calcium, Vitamin D, and protein. However, it's also high in calories, especially full fat milk, so it's important to choose low-fat milk or limit the amount consumed.

It's important to remember that weight loss is not just about what you eat but also about your overall lifestyle. Making healthy food choices, regular physical activity, and finding ways to manage stress are all important factors in achieving and maintaining a healthy weight.

> ### Is soup and bread for dinner time is fine for month?

Soup and bread for dinner every night for a month may not provide a balanced and varied diet. Soup and bread can be a healthy dinner option, but it may not provide adequate amount of essential nutrients such as protein, vitamins and minerals, and healthy fats.

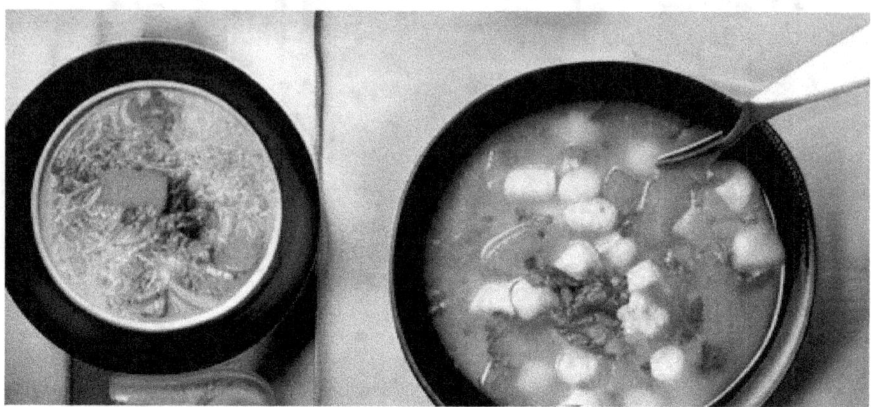

Bread is mostly carbohydrates and it is not a good source of protein, which is important to repair and build muscle and other body tissue.

Soup can be a good source of hydration and some vitamins and minerals, but it depends on the ingredients of the soup. A healthy soup should include a variety of vegetables and a lean protein source such as chicken, fish, or legumes.

It's essential to include a variety of different food groups in your diet, including fruits, vegetables, whole grains, lean protein, and healthy fats. It is always best to consult a healthcare professional or a registered dietitian before making any significant changes to your diet.

It's also worth noting that eating the same thing every night might become monotonous and could lead to feelings of disinterest in food, which can cause problems with adherence to the diet.

➤ **Is eating only banana for dinner reduce weight?**

Eating only bananas for dinner, or any other meal, is not a sustainable or healthy way to lose weight. A diet that consists of only one food or food group is not balanced and will not provide adequate nutrition.

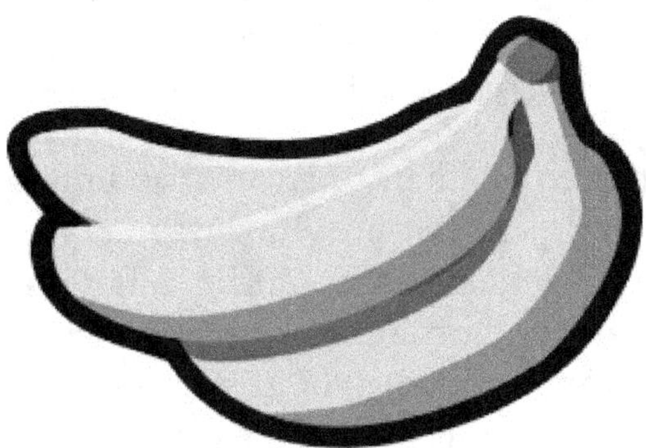

Bananas are a healthy food and can be part of a weight loss diet, as they are low in calories and high in fiber, vitamins, and minerals. However, they alone do not provide a balanced and varied diet and will not provide enough essential nutrients such as protein, healthy fats, and other vitamins and minerals.

A calorie deficit is necessary for weight loss. But it's important to achieve it through a balanced diet that provides all the essential nutrients, and not by eating just one type of food. Additionally, it can lead to feelings of disinterest in food, which can cause problems with adherence to the diet, and also lead to disordered eating.

It's important to consult a healthcare professional or a registered dietitian before making any significant changes to your diet, specially if you're planning to lose weight. They can help you design a safe and healthy weight loss plan that includes a balanced diet and regular physical activity.

> ### Is eating just fruit salad for one week reduce weight?

Eating only a fruit salad for one week may cause weight loss, as fruit is generally low in calories and high in fiber, vitamins, and minerals. However, it is not a balanced or sustainable way to lose weight.

A diet that consists of only one food or food group, such as a fruit salad, will not provide adequate nutrition, and it can lead to deficiencies in essential nutrients such as protein, healthy fats, and other vitamins and minerals. Additionally, it can lead to feelings of disinterest in food, which can cause problems with adherence to the diet, and also lead to disordered eating.

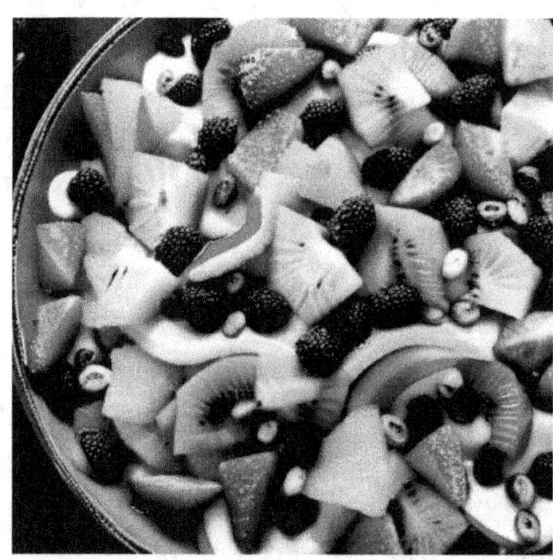

Fruits are a great addition to a weight loss diet, as they are low in calories and high in nutrients, but they should be consumed as part of a balanced diet that includes a variety of different food groups, including fruits, vegetables, whole grains, lean protein, and healthy fats.

It's important to consult a healthcare professional or a

registered dietitian before making any significant changes to your diet, especially if you're planning to lose weight. They can help you design a safe and healthy weight loss plan that includes a balanced diet and regular physical activity. And also, it's important to remember that weight loss is not just about what you eat but also about your overall lifestyle. Making healthy food choices, regular physical activity, and finding ways to manage stress are all important factors in achieving and maintaining a healthy weight.

➢ **Is eating vegetable salad, egg and some seeds like chickpeas and moong beans are fine for dinner to reduce weight?**
Eating a vegetable salad, eggs and some seeds like chickpeas and moong beans for dinner can be a healthy and balanced option for weight loss.

Vegetable salad is low in calories and high in fiber, vitamins and minerals, they provide hydration and help to fill you up. Eggs are a good source of protein, vitamins and minerals. Chickpeas and moong beans are also good sources of protein and healthy carbohydrates, and they are a good alternative to meat as a source of protein.

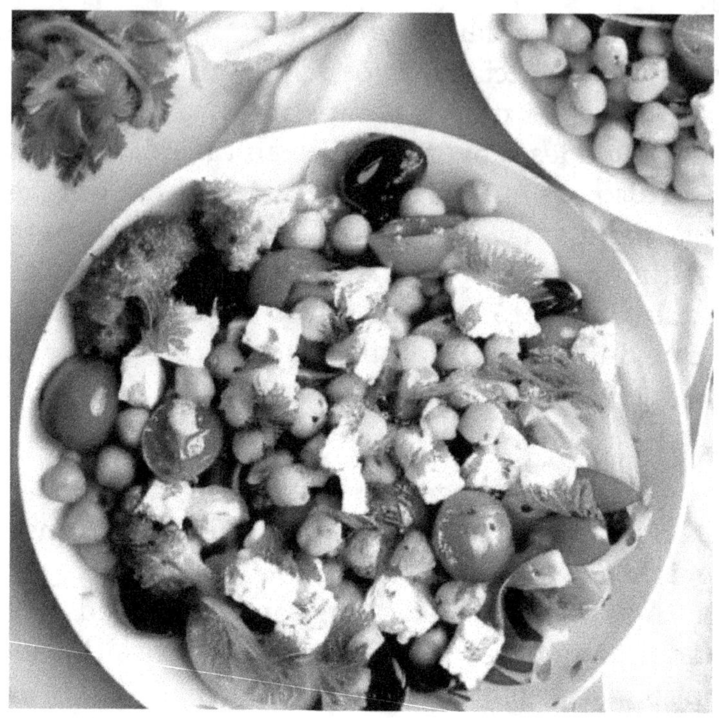

A diet that includes a variety of different food groups, including fruits, vegetables, whole grains, lean protein, and healthy fats is essential for weight loss and overall health. It's important to remember that weight loss is not just about what you eat but also about your overall lifestyle. Making healthy food choices, regular physical activity, and finding ways to manage stress are all important factors in achieving and maintaining a healthy weight.

It's always best to consult a healthcare professional or a registered dietitian before making any significant changes to your diet, especially if you're planning to lose weight. They can help you design a safe and healthy weight loss plan that includes a balanced diet and regular physical activity, taking into account your specific needs and health status.

> **Is it good to eat a Burger every day to lose weight?**

Eating burgers daily is not a healthy or sustainable way to lose weight. While reducing calorie intake is a key factor in weight loss, relying solely on burgers can lead to an unbalanced diet lacking in essential nutrients.

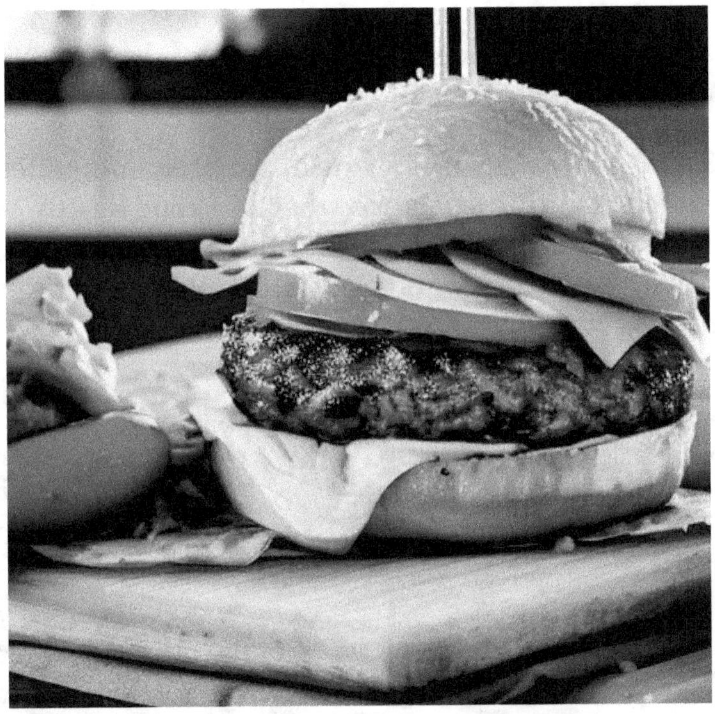

Burgers are often high in calories, fat, and sodium, which can contribute to weight gain and negative health effects when consumed in excess. Additionally, consuming fast food daily can increase the risk of chronic health conditions such as heart disease, high blood pressure, and type 2 diabetes.

To achieve and maintain a healthy weight, it is recommended to have a balanced diet that includes a variety of whole foods, such as fruits, vegetables, whole grains, and lean proteins. Incorporating regular physical activity, reducing stress, and getting enough sleep can also contribute to successful weight loss and overall health.

In summary, eating burgers daily is not a recommended approach for weight loss and can have negative impacts on health. A balanced diet and lifestyle habits are key to maintaining a healthy weight and overall well-being.

> **Is eating Pizza every day good for your health?**

Eating pizza daily is not a healthy or recommended approach for maintaining a balanced diet and good health. While pizza can be a delicious treat, consuming it on a daily basis can lead to excessive calorie and nutrient intake, potentially resulting in weight gain and negative health effects.

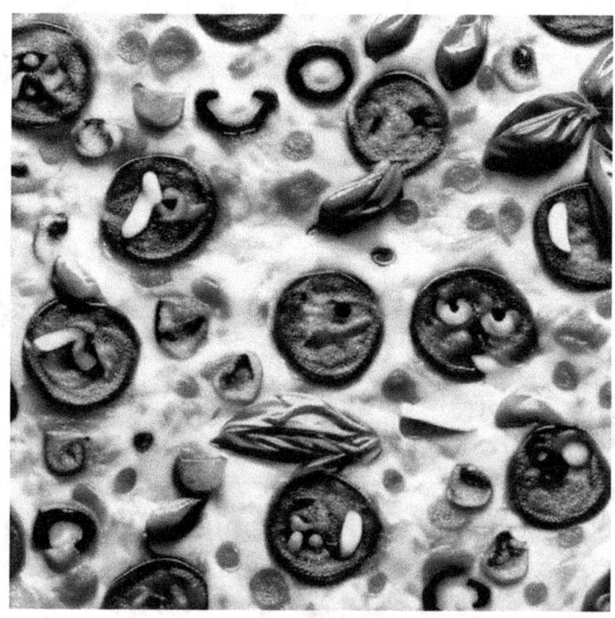

Pizza is often high in calories, fat, and sodium, which can contribute to weight gain and increase the risk of chronic health conditions such as heart disease, high blood pressure, and type 2 diabetes. Additionally, many types of pizza contain refined carbohydrates, which can cause spikes in blood sugar levels and lead to insulin resistance over time.

To maintain a healthy diet, it is recommended to consume a variety of whole foods, such as fruits, vegetables, whole grains, and lean proteins. Incorporating these foods into meals and snacks can help provide essential nutrients and help regulate calorie intake, leading to overall better health.

Incorporating physical activity, reducing stress, and getting enough sleep can also play important roles in maintaining good health. Regular exercise can help control weight, improve cardiovascular health, and support overall physical and mental well-being.

While pizza can be enjoyed in moderation as part of a balanced diet, it is not recommended to consume it daily. Doing so can lead to excessive calorie and nutrient intake, potentially contributing to weight gain and negative health effects.

In summary, eating pizza daily is not a healthy approach for maintaining a balanced diet and good health. It is recommended to incorporate a variety of whole foods, along with regular physical activity, stress reduction, and adequate sleep, for overall well-being.

➤ What is junk food and how does it affect health?

Junk food is a term used to describe food that is high in calories, unhealthy fats, added sugars, and/or sodium but low in essential nutrients such as vitamins, minerals, and fiber. Examples of junk food include fast food, sugary drinks, candy, potato chips, and other processed snack foods.

The consumption of junk food can have negative effects on health, leading to a range of health issues over time. Some of the most significant health effects of consuming junk food include:

Weight gain: Junk food is often high in calories and unhealthy fats, which can contribute to weight gain and obesity. This can increase the risk of chronic health conditions such as heart disease, type 2 diabetes, and certain types of cancer.

Poor nutrition: Junk food is often low in essential nutrients, such as vitamins, minerals, and fiber. This can lead to nutrient deficiencies over time and negatively impact overall health.

Increased risk of chronic health conditions: Regular consumption of junk food has been linked to an increased risk of chronic health conditions such as heart disease, type 2 diabetes, and certain types of cancer.

Negative impact on mental health: Junk food can have a negative impact on mental health, contributing to feelings of guilt and low self-esteem. It can also lead to a cycle of binge eating and yo-yo dieting, which can have long-term effects on mental health.
Poor dental health: Junk food is often high in sugar, which can increase the risk of tooth decay and gum disease.

In addition to these health effects, consuming junk food can also displace healthier food choices and negatively impact overall diet quality. To maintain a healthy diet, it is recommended to limit the consumption of junk food and choose healthier food options instead.

To improve overall health, it is recommended to consume a balanced diet that includes a variety of whole foods, such as fruits, vegetables, whole grains, and lean proteins. Incorporating physical activity, reducing stress, and getting enough sleep can also play important roles in maintaining good health.

In conclusion, junk food is a term used to describe food that is high in calories, unhealthy fats, added sugars, and sodium but low in essential nutrients. Consuming junk food can have negative effects on health, including weight gain, poor nutrition, increased risk of chronic health conditions, negative impact on mental health, and poor dental health. To maintain a healthy diet and good health, it is recommended to limit the consumption of junk food and choose healthier food options instead.

➤ **Can you give some examples of junk foods and how many calories they contain?**

here are some examples of popular junk foods and the approximate calorie content per serving:

French fries: A medium serving of French fries (about 3.5 ounces) contains approximately 365 calories.
Soft drinks: A 12-ounce can of regular soft drink contains approximately 140 calories.

Candy bars: A 1.5-ounce candy bar contains approximately 215 calories.

Chips: A 1-ounce serving of potato chips contains approximately 150 calories.

Burgers: A fast food cheeseburger can contain upwards of

500 calories.

Fried chicken: A 3-piece serving of fried chicken can contain approximately 600 calories.

Ice cream: A 1/2 cup serving of ice cream can contain approximately 150-200 calories.

It is important to note that the calorie content of junk food can vary greatly depending on the type of food and the portion size consumed. Additionally, many junk foods contain added sugars, unhealthy fats, and sodium, which can contribute to weight gain, chronic health conditions, and other negative health effects.

While junk food can be a tempting and delicious treat, consuming it on a regular basis can have negative effects on health. To maintain a healthy diet, it is recommended to limit the consumption of junk food and choose healthier food options instead.
Incorporating a variety of whole foods, such as fruits, vegetables, whole grains, and lean proteins, into meals and snacks can help provide essential nutrients and help regulate calorie intake, leading to overall better health. Incorporating physical activity, reducing stress, and getting enough sleep can also play important roles in maintaining good health.

In conclusion, junk food can contain a high amount of calories and unhealthy nutrients. Examples of junk food include French fries, soft drinks, candy bars, chips, burgers, fried chicken, and ice cream. To maintain a healthy diet and good health, it is recommended to limit the consumption of junk food and choose healthier food options instead.

➤ **Does alcohol or smoking affect weight loss?**

Alcohol and smoking can negatively impact weight loss efforts. Here's how:

Alcohol: Alcohol is high in calories, with an average of 7 calories per gram. Drinking alcohol can lead to an increase in calorie consumption, making it difficult to maintain a calorie deficit, which is necessary for weight loss. In addition, alcohol can impair judgment and lead to overeating or choosing high-calorie foods.

Smoking: Smoking can lead to weight loss, but it is not a healthy way to lose weight. Smoking can suppress appetite and increase metabolism, leading to weight loss. However, the health effects of smoking far outweigh any potential weight loss benefits. In addition, weight gain is common after quitting smoking, as the metabolism returns to normal and appetite increases.

It is important to note that the effects of alcohol and smoking on weight loss will vary depending on individual factors such as metabolism, diet, and physical activity. Maintaining a healthy diet and incorporating physical activity are essential for successful weight loss.

In conclusion, while alcohol and smoking can have some impact on weight, they are not recommended as methods for weight loss due to their negative health effects. Maintaining a healthy diet and incorporating physical activity are more effective and safer methods for weight loss.

➤ Is eating meat good for losing weight?

Eating meat can be a part of a healthy weight loss diet, but it depends on the type of meat and how it is prepared. Here are some considerations:

Protein: Meat is a good source of protein, which can help with weight loss by increasing feelings of fullness and reducing hunger. Higher protein diets have been shown to be more effective for weight loss compared to diets lower in protein.

Fat content: The fat content of meat can vary greatly, with some cuts being high in unhealthy saturated fats and others being lower in fat. Choosing lean cuts of meat, such as chicken breast or turkey, can help keep calorie and fat intake in check.

Cooking methods: The way meat is prepared can also affect its calorie content. For example, frying meat in oil can add extra calories, while grilling or baking meat can help reduce calorie intake.

However, it is important to note that eating too much meat, especially processed meats such as bacon and sausages, can be harmful to health and may contribute to weight gain. Processed meats are often high in sodium, unhealthy fats, and preservatives, which can increase the risk of chronic health conditions such as heart disease and cancer.

In conclusion, eating meat can be a part of a healthy weight loss diet, but it is important to choose lean cuts of meat and prepare them in a healthy way. Incorporating a variety of protein sources, including plant-based proteins, can help provide essential nutrients and support weight loss efforts. It is also important to limit the consumption of processed meats and choose healthier protein options instead.

➤ **Chicken, fish, beef or lamb, what helps you lose weight?**

All meats can be a part of a weight loss diet, but the best choice for weight loss will depend on several factors, including:

Protein content: All meats are good sources of protein, which can help with weight loss by increasing feelings of fullness and reducing hunger.

Fat content: Chicken and fish are generally lower in fat compared to beef and lamb, making them a better choice for those looking to lose weight. However, it's important to choose lean cuts of meat, regardless of the type, and remove any visible fat.

Cooking methods: The way meat is prepared can also affect its calorie content. For example, frying meat in oil can add extra calories, while grilling or baking meat can help reduce calorie intake.

In conclusion, all meats can be a part of a weight loss diet, but chicken and fish are generally lower in fat and may be a better choice for those looking to lose weight. Regardless of the type of meat, it's important to choose lean cuts and prepare them in a healthy way to support weight loss efforts. It is also important to incorporate a variety of protein sources, including plant-based proteins, to provide essential nutrients and support overall health.

➤ **Is drinking coffee good for weight loss?**

When it comes to weight loss and coffee, there is a lot of confusion about the potential benefits and risks. On the one hand, coffee does contain some compounds that may have a slight positive effect on fat burning and metabolism, but on the other hand, drinking too much coffee can lead to dehydration and poor eating habits, both of which can have a negative impact on weight loss efforts.

At the end of the day, the best approach is to find a healthy balance. Coffee can be a part of a weight loss plan if consumed in moderation, but it is important to keep an eye on your overall caffeine intake throughout the day.

For starters, it is recommended that adults consume no more than 400 mg of caffeine per day. That works out to roughly four 8-ounce cups of coffee. Any more than that can lead to side effects such as jitters, headaches, and insomnia. It is important to stay within this range to reduce the risk of these effects.

When it comes to coffee and weight loss, the key is to drink it in moderation and to ensure that you are drinking the right type. For example, black coffee with no added sugars or creams is a much better choice than a latte or mocha which can be loaded with calories. Also, adding cream and sugar can increase the overall calorie count of your coffee drink, so it is important to be aware of this when choosing a beverage.

Finally, it is important to remember that coffee is not a replacement for a healthy diet or exercise. In order to see results, it is important to combine a balanced diet and regular physical activity with moderate coffee consumption. This approach can help you achieve the desired weight loss results.

➤ **Should we know the nutritional plan and follow it continuously, or should a one-off nutritional plan provide a lasting result?**

The best way to achieve a desired body shape is to have a

balanced and consistent approach to eating and exercise. A one-time diet plan may give you short-term results, but it is unlikely to provide you with long-term success. To maintain the results of any diet, you must make permanent changes to your lifestyle.

One way to begin is by setting realistic goals. To make sure you stick to your plan, start by gradually changing your diet and exercising habits. Focus on small, achievable goals that can be easily incorporated into your lifestyle. Make sure your meals are balanced, incorporating all the food groups, and that your portions are appropriate for your body type and activity level.

In addition to diet and exercise, you should also ensure that you get enough sleep and rest. Adequate amounts of sleep are essential to keep your body in top shape and maintain your focus for the day. Additionally, create a routine that can help you stick to your goals. Schedule specific activities at a certain time of day and reward yourself for achieving them.

Creating healthy habits is the most effective way to reach your desired weight. Eating a balanced diet and exercising regularly should become an essential part of your daily routine in order to keep the weight off. Additionally, make sure to stay hydrated and consume plenty of fiber, as these can help you stay full and reduce cravings.

Finally, it's important to remember that no one diet plan is right for everyone. Everyone's body is different and may need different strategies to reach their goals. Find a plan that works for you and be consistent with it in order to achieve the best results in the long-term.

Chapter Summary/Key Takeaways:

In conclusion, this chapter has discussed the various types of foods that can be incorporated into a weight loss plan. We highlighted the importance of a balanced diet that includes a variety of nutrient-dense foods such as fruits, vegetables, whole grains, lean proteins, and healthy fats. We also discussed the benefits of certain foods such as high-fiber foods and protein-rich foods, which can help with weight loss by promoting feelings of fullness and supporting muscle growth.

We also touched on the concept of calorie-dense and calorie-light foods. And how choosing foods that are lower in calories but still provide essential nutrients can help you lose weight without feeling deprived. Additionally, we discussed the benefits of avoiding processed foods and added sugars, which can be high in calories and contribute to weight gain.

It's important to remember that weight loss is not about restriction, it's about finding the balance between calorie intake and calorie expenditure. And creating a diet plan that works for you and your lifestyle. Remember that weight loss is a process and it's not always easy, it's okay to have setbacks and slip-ups, the important thing is to get back on track and don't give up. With the right plan and the right mindset, you can achieve your weight loss goals and improve your overall health and well-being.

In the previous chapter, we discussed the importance of incorporating nutrient-dense foods into your weight loss plan and the benefits of certain foods such as high-fiber foods and protein-rich foods. We also touched on the concept of calorie-dense and calorie-light foods and the importance of avoiding processed foods and added sugars.

In this next chapter, we will shift our focus to the role of exercise in weight loss. Just as a balanced diet is crucial for weight loss, regular physical activity is essential for burning calories and building muscle. We will discuss the different types of exercises that can be included in a weight loss plan and how to create an exercise routine that is both effective and sustainable.

Exercise not only helps with weight loss but also improve overall health, including cardiovascular health and mental health. We will also talk about how to overcome common exercise barriers and how to make exercise enjoyable. We will explore the different types of exercises, from high-intensity interval training to resistance training, and we will explain how they can benefit weight loss.

In short, exercise and nutrition are both important parts of a weight loss plan, and both have to work hand in hand. In this chapter, we will explore the different types of exercises that can be included in a weight loss plan and how to create an exercise routine that is both effective and sustainable.

7. EXERCISES TO LOSE WEIGHT

Exercise is one of the most important components of a healthy lifestyle. It not only helps people achieve and maintain physical fitness, but it also has the potential to improve mental health. Exercise can help people lose weight and keep it off through burning calories, building muscle, and increasing metabolism.

When looking to lose weight, it is important to find an exercise plan that is tailored to the individual's needs and goals. For example, someone who is looking to shed a few pounds may want to focus on low impact exercises such as swimming, walking, or yoga. For those looking to build muscle, resistance training such as weight-lifting might be more beneficial. Additionally, interval training, where bouts of high-intensity exercise are alternated with short rest periods, can help to boost metabolism and burn more calories.

Regular exercise can also help to prevent weight gain. Studies have shown that physical activity can help to reduce fat storage and promote a healthier metabolism. In the long-term, this can help to prevent the accumulation of excess body fat. Exercise can also help to improve the body's ability to respond to insulin and reduce the risk of developing metabolic diseases. Exercise also provides psychological benefits, including improved mood and increased self-esteem. Along with helping to reduce stress and anxiety, exercise can also provide a sense of accomplishment and satisfaction. This can help to motivate individuals to stick to a fitness plan and achieve their weight loss goals.

In conclusion, exercising can be an important component of any weight loss plan. While it can help to burn calories and build muscle, it can also provide psychological benefits. Exercise should be tailored to the individual's needs and goals and should be performed regularly for maximum benefit.

7.1. Popular Exercises
to Lose Weight

Exercise can be an important component of weight loss, as it helps to burn calories and build muscle. There are many different types of exercise that can be effective for weight loss, and the best exercise for you will depend on your current fitness level, preferences, and goals. Here are some examples of exercises that can be helpful for weight loss:

Cardio exercises: Cardio exercises, such as running, cycling, swimming, or dancing, are great for burning calories and improving cardiovascular fitness.

These exercises work by increasing your heart rate and making you sweat, which helps to burn calories and fat. Some of the most popular cardio exercises include running, cycling, swimming, jumping rope, and using an elliptical machine.

Running is a high-impact exercise that can be done almost anywhere and is an excellent way to build cardiovascular endurance. Cycling is a low-impact exercise that is easy on your joints and can be done indoors or outdoors. Swimming is another low-impact exercise that is great for those with joint pain or injuries. Jumping rope is a high-intensity exercise that can be done anywhere and is a fun way to burn calories. Using an elliptical machine is a low-impact exercise that provides an intense cardiovascular workout.

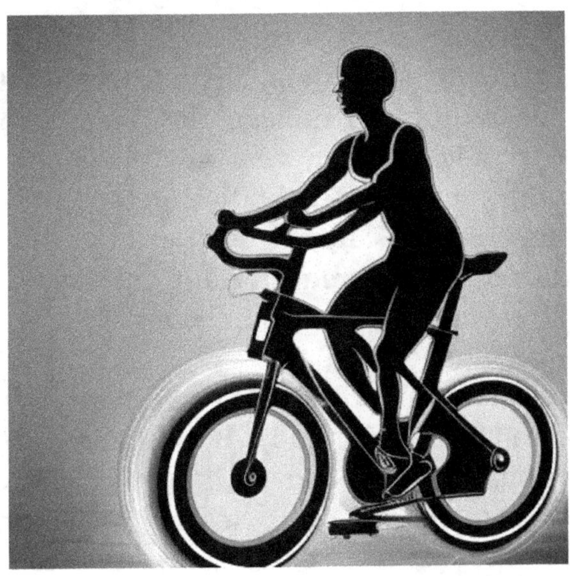

Regardless of which cardio exercise you choose, it's important to start slow and gradually increase the intensity and duration of your workouts. To maximize the benefits of cardio exercises for weight loss, it's recommended to perform these exercises for at least 30 minutes, three to four times per week.

It's also important to keep in mind that cardio exercises are just one part of an overall healthy lifestyle. Eating a balanced diet that is rich in fruits, vegetables, and lean protein can help support your weight loss goals. Additionally, incorporating strength training exercises into your routine can help build muscle, which can increase your metabolism and help you burn even more calories.

To lose weight, cardio exercises such as running, cycling, swimming, or dancing should be done for at least 30 minutes a day, at least 5 days a week. However, to see significant weight loss results, it is recommended to engage in cardio exercises for longer periods of time, such as 45-60 minutes a day, or even up to several hours a day for more intense endurance activities like marathon training.

Strength training: Strength training, such as weight lifting, bodyweight exercises, or resistance band exercises, can help to build muscle and increase metabolism. Strength training is a crucial aspect of weight loss and can play a major role in helping individuals to achieve their fitness goals. By building muscle, strength training increases the body's metabolic rate, which in turn helps to burn more calories even at rest. This means that individuals who engage in strength training will continue to burn calories long after their workout is finished.

In addition to increasing metabolism, strength training also helps to tone and shape the body. By targeting specific muscle groups, individuals can work towards a more defined physique, giving them a more aesthetically pleasing appearance. This can help to boost confidence and self-esteem, which is important for individuals who are looking to lose weight.

There are several ways to incorporate strength training into a weight loss program, including using weightlifting equipment such as dumbbells or barbells, using resistance bands, or bodyweight exercises such as push-ups and squats. It is important to use proper form and technique when engaging in strength training exercises to reduce the risk of injury and ensure that the body is working in the most efficient way possible.

For those new to strength training, it is important to start slowly and gradually increase the weight or resistance being used. This will help to build muscle and strength in a safe and effective way. Additionally, it is important to engage in a well-rounded fitness program that includes both strength training and cardiovascular exercise. This will help to maximize the benefits of weight loss and improve overall health and well-being.

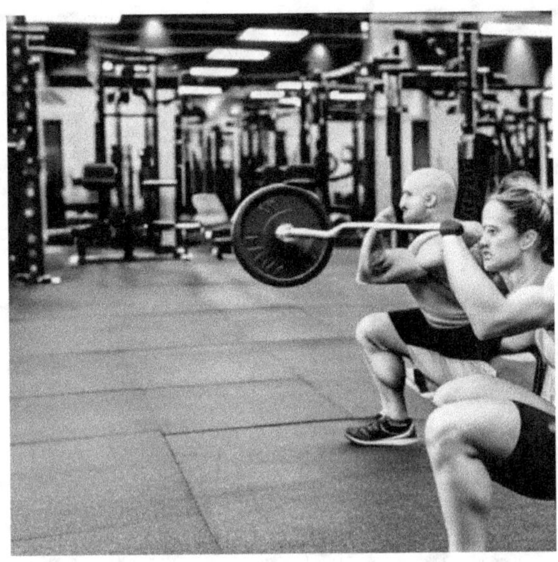

In conclusion, strength training can be an extremely effective tool for weight loss. By increasing metabolism and building muscle, individuals can achieve their weight loss goals and create a healthier, more toned body. When incorporated into a well-rounded fitness program, strength training can help to achieve optimal health and wellness. Strength training exercises such as weight lifting, bodyweight exercises, or resistance band exercises should be done at least 2-3 times a week for 30-45 minutes per session.

High-Intensity Interval Training (HIIT): HIIT is a type of cardio that alternates short periods of intense activity with periods of recovery. It is a highly effective way to burn calories and improve cardiovascular fitness.

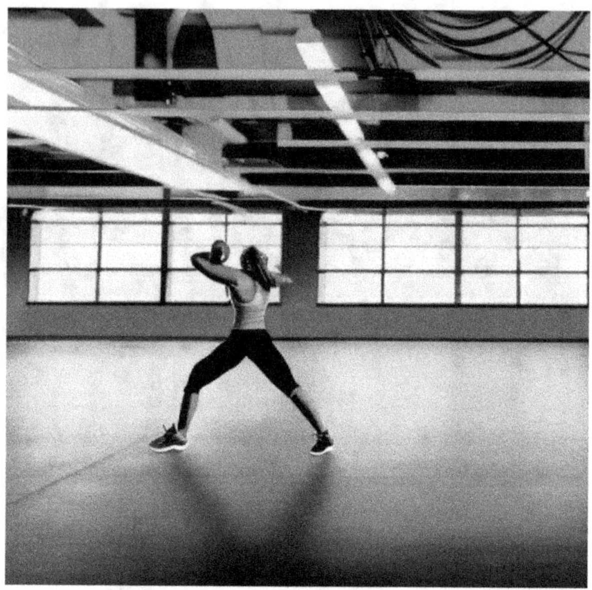

High-Intensity Interval Training (HIIT) is a type of workout that has become increasingly popular for weight loss. It involves alternating periods of high-intensity exercise with periods of rest or low-intensity exercise. This type of workout is known for its ability to burn a high number of calories in a short amount of time, making it an ideal choice for individuals looking to lose weight.

One of the key benefits of HIIT is that it can increase the body's metabolic rate for several hours after the workout is finished. This means that individuals will continue to burn calories even after their workout is completed, making it an effective tool for weight loss. In addition, HIIT can help to build lean muscle, which in turn helps to increase the body's metabolism, making it easier to lose weight and maintain a healthy weight.

When engaging in HIIT, it is important to choose exercises that are high-intensity and challenging, such as running, jumping, or plyometrics. This will help to maximize the benefits of the workout and improve overall fitness. Additionally, it is important to vary the exercises used in HIIT to target different muscle groups and keep the body guessing, leading to better results.

HIIT is a great choice for individuals who are short on time, as it allows for a highly effective workout in just a few minutes. This makes it an ideal choice for those who are busy and have limited time for exercise. Additionally, HIIT can be easily modified to fit the individual's fitness level, making it a great choice for people of all fitness levels and abilities.

In conclusion, HIIT is an excellent choice for individuals who are looking to lose weight. With its ability to increase the body's metabolism and build lean muscle, HIIT can help individuals to achieve their weight loss goals quickly and effectively. When incorporated into a well-rounded fitness program, HIIT can help to improve overall health and wellness.

High-Intensity Interval Training (HIIT) should be done 2-3 times a week for 20-30 minutes per session.

Yoga and Pilates: These types of exercises focus on building core strength and flexibility, they can also help to reduce stress and improve mental health. Yoga and Pilates are two low-impact forms of exercise that have become increasingly popular for weight loss. Both practices offer a variety of benefits that can help individuals to achieve their weight loss goals, making them an excellent addition to a well-rounded fitness program.

Yoga is a practice that focuses on mindfulness, breath control, and physical postures. It has been shown to help reduce stress and improve flexibility, which can in turn lead to weight loss. By incorporating mindfulness and breathing techniques into the workout, individuals can learn to better control their eating habits, making it easier to maintain a healthy weight. Additionally, many yoga poses involve strengthening and stretching the muscles, which can help to build lean muscle and boost metabolism, making it easier to lose weight.

Pilates, like yoga, is a low-impact form of exercise that focuses on strengthening and stretching the muscles. It has been shown to help improve posture, balance, and flexibility, which can lead to weight loss. Additionally, Pilates can help to build lean muscle, which in turn boosts the body's metabolism, making it easier to lose weight. Pilates exercises often use resistance from springs or bands, making it possible to target specific muscle groups and achieve a more toned appearance.

When incorporating yoga and Pilates into a weight loss program, it is important to choose a class that is challenging and that focuses on proper form and technique. This will help to maximize the benefits of the workout and ensure that the body is working in the most efficient way possible. Additionally, it is important to engage in a well-rounded fitness program that includes both yoga and Pilates as well as other forms of exercise such as cardiovascular exercise and strength training.

In conclusion, yoga and Pilates are two excellent choices for individuals who are looking to lose weight. With their ability to reduce stress, improve posture, and build lean muscle, both practices can help individuals to achieve their weight loss goals and improve overall health and wellness. When incorporated into a well-rounded fitness program, yoga and Pilates can provide a comprehensive approach to weight loss and help individuals to achieve their fitness goals.

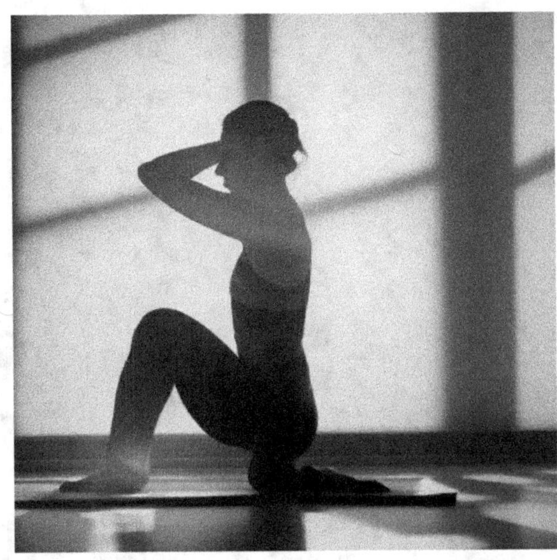

Yoga and Pilates should be done 2-3 times a week for 30-45 minutes per session.

Outdoor activities:

Activities such as hiking, rock climbing,and kayaking can be a fun and effective way to lose weight and get in shape.
Outdoor activities such as hiking, rock climbing, and kayaking should be done for at least 30-60 minutes a day, at least 3-4 days a week. It's important to note that these times are general recommendations and the optimal duration of exercise will vary depending on an individual's goals, fitness level and overall health status.

And also, It's important to maintain a healthy diet and get enough sleep to help support weight loss efforts. Outdoor activities provide a fun and invigorating way to lose weight and improve overall health.

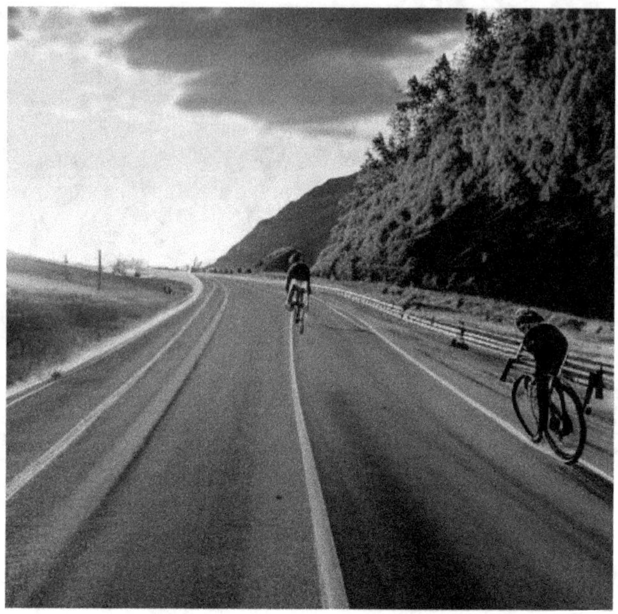

From walking and running to hiking and cycling, the great outdoors offers numerous options for physical activity.

Walking and running are simple and accessible ways to burn calories and lose weight. Going for a walk or run in the park or on the beach can provide a change of scenery from the gym and help reduce stress levels.

Hiking is another great outdoor activity that can help burn calories and build muscle. Whether you're trekking through the mountains or exploring a nature trail, hiking can be a challenging and rewarding workout. The uneven terrain and steep inclines can also provide an added cardiovascular challenge that can help increase weight loss.

Cycling is another outdoor activity that can aid in weight loss. Whether you're riding on a road or mountain bike, cycling provides an excellent cardiovascular workout that can help burn calories and improve overall fitness.

Swimming is another fun outdoor activity that can aid in weight loss. Swimming is a low-impact exercise that can provide a full-body workout and burn a significant number of calories. Whether you're swimming laps or simply splashing around, swimming can provide a fun and invigorating workout.

Stand-up paddleboarding (SUP) is a relatively new outdoor activity that is growing in popularity. SUP provides a low-impact workout that can be performed on calm waters, making it a fun and challenging way to burn calories and improve fitness.

Finally, playing outdoor sports such as basketball, tennis, and soccer can be an enjoyable way to get moving and lose weight. Not only do these sports provide a fun and competitive workout, but they also require quick movements and coordination, which can help build muscle and increase weight loss.

In conclusion, there are many outdoor activities that can be useful in losing weight and improving overall health. Whether you prefer a leisurely walk, a challenging hike, or a competitive sport, the great outdoors offers numerous options for physical activity that can provide a fun and invigorating workout.

It's important to note that it's important to have a balance of cardio, strength training, and flexibility in your workout routine, to target all your muscles, and to avoid boredom. Additionally, it's important to consult with a doctor or a trainer before starting a new exercise program, especially if you have any health conditions.

Planning Your Exercises:

Set a goal: Decide how much weight you want to lose and set a specific, measurable goal. This goal should be realistic and attainable, and should take into account factors such as your current weight, body composition, and overall health. For example, a goal to lose 1-2 pounds per week is considered safe and healthy.

Assess your fitness level: Determine your current fitness level by taking into account your age, health, and current activity level. This will help you determine what type of exercise is appropriate for you. If you are new to exercise or have any health conditions, it's important to consult with a healthcare professional before starting an exercise program.

Create a schedule: Plan out a schedule that includes the types of exercise you want to do, the days of the week, and the times of day that work best for you. Make sure to include a mix of cardio, strength training, and flexibility exercises. Cardio exercises such as running, cycling, swimming, or dancing should be done for at least 30 minutes a day, at least 5 days a week. Strength training exercises such as weight lifting, bodyweight exercises, or resistance band exercises should be done at least 2-3 times a week for 30-45 minutes per session.

Be consistent: Stick to your schedule as much as possible. Consistency is key when it comes to losing weight through exercise. It's important to make exercise a regular part of your daily routine.

Track your progress: Keep track of your progress by measuring your weight, body fat percentage, and measurements, as well as by noting how you feel. This will help you see whether your exercise program is working and make adjustments as needed.

Adjust as necessary: If you're not seeing the results you want, adjust your exercise program to include more intense or longer workouts, or add more days of exercise per week. It's important to keep challenging your body to see progress.

Seek professional help: Consult with a personal trainer or a registered dietitian to help you design a safe and effective exercise program. They can help you to set appropriate goals and tailor a program that meets your specific needs.

Listen to your body: Pay attention to how your body feels during and after exercise, and make adjustments as needed. If you feel unwell or experience pain, stop the exercise and consult with your doctor. It's important to avoid over-exertion and to take rest days as needed.

In addition to the above steps, it is important to maintain a healthy diet, and get enough sleep to help support weight loss efforts. Remember that losing weight is a gradual process, and it is important to be patient with yourself. The most important thing is to stay consistent with your exercise program, and to make adjustments as needed to ensure that you are on track to achieve your goals.

Myths About Exercises When Losing Weight:

When it comes to losing weight, the amount of conflicting information out there can be overwhelming. Many people have developed a wide range of myths about exercises when trying to shed those extra pounds. Here are some of the most common myths about exercises when losing weight.

Myth 1: Engaging in Long Workouts is the Best Way to Lose Weight

This is one of the most pervasive myths about exercises when attempting to lose weight. The truth is that long workouts don't necessarily lead to better results when it comes to losing weight. In fact, shorter bursts of intense exercise are often more effective for weight loss than long stretches of moderate exercise.

Myth 2: You Need to Exercise Constantly in Order to Lose Weight

This is simply not true. While engaging in regular physical activity is important for weight management, it is not necessary to exercise at all hours of the day in order to lose weight. Instead, it is important to focus on finding a sustainable exercise routine that fits into your lifestyle and can be easily maintained day after day.

Myth 3: You Don't Need to Watch Your Diet if You Exercise

Another myth about exercises when trying to lose weight is that you don't need to watch your diet if you are engaging in regular physical activity. This is far from true. While exercise is important for weight management, it is also necessary to have a healthy and balanced diet in order to maximize weight loss.

Myth 4: All Exercises are Equal When it Comes to Weight Loss

It is a common misconception that all exercises are equally beneficial for weight loss. In reality, different types of activity have different effects on the body. For example, activities like running and cycling can burn a significant number of calories, whereas activities like yoga and Pilates are better for toning and improving posture. Therefore, it is important to tailor your exercise routine to your specific goals.

Myth 5: You Can Lose Weight Without Exercising

This is something that many people believe, but unfortunately it is not true. Exercising is an essential part of any weight loss program, as it helps to burn off excess calories and provides a wide range of health benefits. Therefore, it is important to make sure that you are engaging in regular physical activity in order to maximize your weight loss results.

Overall, it is important to be aware of the myths about exercises when trying to lose:

7.2. Issues / Problems and how to overcome them

Exercise is an essential part of maintaining a healthy lifestyle, but it's not always easy. Several problems can arise when attempting to start or maintain an exercise routine, but with the right approach, these issues can be overcome.

One of the most common problems is a lack of motivation. It can be challenging to find the energy and drive to exercise, especially when starting a new routine. Overcoming this issue requires finding a source of inspiration and setting achievable goals. Surrounding oneself with supportive friends and family, or finding a workout buddy, can also provide the motivation needed to stick to an exercise routine.

Another common problem is injury. Engaging in physical activity can put stress on the body, and if proper form and technique are not used, injury can occur. To avoid injury, it's essential to warm up and cool down properly, use proper form and technique, and listen to your body when it signals that it's time to rest. Seeking the advice of a trainer or physical therapist can also help reduce the risk of injury.

Time constraints can also be an issue when attempting to exercise. With busy schedules, it can be challenging to find time to work out. Overcoming this issue requires scheduling exercise into one's daily routine and making it a priority. Finding exercises that can be done at home or during the workday can also help maximize time and increase the likelihood of sticking to an exercise routine.

Finally, boredom is another common problem when exercising.

Doing the same workout routine day after day can become monotonous, leading to a loss of motivation. To overcome this issue, it's essential to switch up your routine, try new exercises, and keep your workout fresh and exciting.

In conclusion, there are several problems that can arise when attempting to start or maintain an exercise routine. However, with the right approach, these issues can be overcome. Finding a source of motivation, avoiding injury, maximizing time, and avoiding boredom are key to sticking to an exercise routine and achieving your goals. Remember, exercise is not just about losing weight but also improving overall health and well-being, so it's essential to make it a priority and stick to it.

Chapter Summary/Key Takeaways

The book chapter provides an overview of different exercises that can be used for weight loss, including cardio, strength training, high-intensity interval training (HIIT), yoga and Pilates, and outdoor activities. The chapter also covers how to plan an exercise program for weight loss, including setting specific, measurable goals and tracking progress.

The chapter also addresses common issues and problems that people may encounter when trying to lose weight through exercise, such as lack of motivation, difficulty sticking to a schedule, not seeing results, pain or injury, plateaus, and boredom. The chapter offers strategies for overcoming these issues, such as finding an activity that is enjoyable, scheduling workouts in advance, increasing the intensity or duration of workouts, and seeking professional help. The chapter emphasizes the importance of being patient with the process of weight loss and making adjustments as needed to achieve one's goals.

The next chapter builds on the information provided in the previous chapter by focusing on how to effectively follow through with an exercise plan for weight loss. This chapter provides practical tips and strategies for staying motivated, staying on track, and making adjustments to the plan as needed. It also covers the importance of consistency and commitment to the plan, and provides strategies for dealing with setbacks and obstacles that may arise.

8. FALLOW YOUR PLAN

It is often said that the best-laid plans are doomed to failure, but that couldn't be further from the truth when it comes to weight loss. Planning is an essential part of any successful weight loss journey, as it helps to keep you on track and accountable. Here are some tips to help you follow your plan and achieve your weight loss goals.

Firstly, aim to make small, achievable goals that are realistic and attainable. For example, if your goal is to lose 10 pounds in the next month, break it down into smaller chunks and aim for 1-2 pounds each week. This will help make it more manageable and help you to stay focused.

Secondly, plan your meals and snacks in advance. Meal planning not only helps you to stay on track with your diet, but it also helps to reduce food waste. Spend some time each week looking up healthy recipes and writing out a meal plan for the week. Planning meals and snacks can also help to reduce your grocery spending.

Thirdly, plan your workouts. Regular exercise is essential for any weight loss plan, but it's important to make sure that you're doing the right kind of exercise, and that you're not over-exerting yourself. If you're new to exercise, try walking or jogging, or look up beginner friendly workouts online.

Finally, don't forget to stay hydrated. Water is essential for any diet, and it can also help to keep you feeling full and curb cravings. Aim to drink at least 8 glasses of water each day.

Following your weight loss plan is essential if you want to achieve your weight loss goals. By setting achievable goals, planning your meals and snacks, planning your workouts and staying hydrated, you will be sure to stay on track and maximize your results. Good luck!

8.1. Following a weight loss plan

In this chapter, we will delve into the importance of following a weight loss plan in order to achieve your desired results. Losing weight is not a one-time event, but rather a lifestyle change that requires commitment and consistency. We will discuss how to set realistic goals, create a plan, and track progress in order to stay motivated and on track. Additionally, we will explore the importance of regular physical activity, making healthy food choices, getting enough sleep, and seeking support from friends, family, and professionals.

However, even with the best intentions, following a weight loss plan can be challenging and it's important to be aware of common issues that arise and how to overcome them. This chapter will provide you with the tools and strategies you need to successfully follow a weight loss plan and reach your weight loss goals.

Following a weight loss plan can be challenging, but it can be done with the right mindset and approach. Here are some tips to help you successfully follow a weight loss plan:

Set realistic goals: Start by setting realistic and achievable goals for yourself. This will help you stay motivated and on track. When setting goals, it's important to focus on a healthy weight loss rate of about 1-2 pounds per week. This can be achieved through a combination of calorie reduction and increased physical activity.

Create a plan: Create a detailed plan that outlines what you will eat, when you will exercise, and how you will track your progress. A plan will help you stay organized and motivated, and make it easier to monitor your progress. Consider breaking down your goals into smaller, manageable steps and set deadlines to keep yourself accountable.

Keep a food journal: Keeping a food journal can help you stay accountable for what you eat and make it easier to identify areas where you may need to make changes. A food journal will allow you to track your calorie intake, as well as the types of foods you are eating. This can help you identify any triggers that may be causing you to overeat or make poor food choices.

Incorporate exercise: Regular physical activity is an essential part of any weight loss plan. Aim to get at least 30 minutes of moderate-intensity exercise most days of the week. This can be achieved through a variety of activities such as running, cycling, swimming, or dancing. Exercise not only burns calories but also helps to boost your metabolism and improve cardiovascular fitness.

Make healthy food choices: Focus on eating nutrient-dense foods that are high in fiber and protein, and low in added sugars and saturated fats. Eating a balanced diet will help you feel full and satisfied, and prevent overeating. Eating more fruits, vegetables, and whole grains can help you feel full without consuming too many calories.

Stay consistent: Weight loss is a gradual process, so it's important to be consistent with your efforts. Don't get discouraged if you slip up or have a bad day, just get back on track the next day. Remember, it's important to be patient and persistent in order to see results.

Stay motivated: Finding ways to stay motivated is essential for long-term success. Surround yourself with supportive friends and family, and consider working with a personal trainer or a nutritionist for additional support. Joining a support group or online community can also be helpful.

Get enough sleep: Getting enough sleep is crucial for weight loss, as well as overall health. Aim for at least 7-8 hours of sleep each night. Lack of sleep can lead to weight gain and a decrease in metabolism, so it's important to prioritize getting enough rest.

Remember, following a weight loss plan is not a one-time thing, it's a lifestyle change. Stay consistent, make healthy food choices, and stay active. It takes time to see results, but with patience and persistence, you'll get there.

8.2. Issues / Problems and how to overcome them

When following a weight loss plan, one of the most common issues people may face is lack of motivation. It can be difficult to stay motivated when progress is slow or when temptations to indulge in unhealthy habits arise. To overcome this issue, it's important to set realistic and achievable goals, and to find ways to stay motivated. This can include surrounding yourself with supportive friends and family, working with a personal trainer or nutritionist, or finding an exercise or activity that you enjoy.

Another common issue is the struggle to stick to a healthy diet. It can be difficult to make healthy food choices, especially when surrounded by tempting and convenient unhealthy options. To overcome this, it's important to plan ahead and have healthy food options readily available. It can also be helpful to keep a food journal to track progress and identify areas where improvements can be made.

Another common issue is lack of consistency. It's easy to fall off track and slip into old habits. To overcome this, it's important to have a plan in place and to stay consistent with efforts. Don't be too hard on yourself if you slip up, just get back on track the next day.

Finally, lack of time can be an issue when trying to incorporate regular exercise and meal planning into a busy schedule. To overcome this, it's important to prioritize and make time for self-care and weight loss efforts. This can include scheduling exercise and meal prep time into a daily or weekly routine, or finding ways to make healthy habits more convenient such as prepping meals for the week on the weekends or finding ways to incorporate physical activity into daily routine like taking the stairs instead of the elevator.

This book chapter focuses on the importance of following a weight loss plan in order to achieve success. The chapter provides tips for setting realistic goals, creating a plan, keeping a food journal, incorporating exercise, making healthy food choices, staying consistent, staying motivated, getting enough sleep, and recognizing that weight loss is a lifestyle change.

The chapter also addresses common issues that can arise when following a weight loss plan, such as lack of motivation, lack of consistency, and difficulty sticking to the plan. To overcome these issues, the chapter suggests finding ways to stay motivated, surrounding oneself with supportive friends and family, and considering working with a personal trainer or nutritionist for additional support.

Additionally, it's important to remember that weight loss is a gradual process and to not get discouraged if progress is slow. With patience and persistence, it's possible to achieve weight loss success.

9. CONCLUSION

In conclusion, weight loss is an important issue for many individuals, as excess weight can lead to a variety of health problems, including heart disease, type 2 diabetes, and certain types of cancer. It is important for individuals who are struggling with their weight to find a solution that works for them, as losing weight can bring about a wide range of benefits, including improved health, increased energy, and increased self-esteem.

When it comes to weight loss, motivation is key. Finding a source of inspiration and setting achievable goals can help individuals to stay on track and achieve their weight loss goals. Additionally, choosing a weight loss plan that is sustainable and fits with individual lifestyle and preferences is essential.

There are many popular diets that can help individuals to lose weight, including low-carb diets, high-protein diets, and low-fat diets. It is important to choose a diet that is balanced and provides the body with all of the nutrients it needs to function properly. Additionally, it is important to choose a diet that is sustainable, as yo-yo dieting can lead to weight gain and other health problems.
In terms of exercise, there are many different forms of exercise that can help individuals to lose weight, including strength training, high-intensity interval training, yoga, and Pilates. It is important to choose a form of exercise that is enjoyable and fits with individual lifestyle and preferences, as this will help to ensure that the individual is able to stick with the exercise plan and achieve their weight loss goals.

When planning a weight loss program, it is important to start with realistic goals and a well-rounded approach that includes a healthy diet and regular exercise. Additionally, it is important to track progress and make adjustments to the plan as needed. Finally, it is important to be patient and not become discouraged if progress is slow.

The amount of weight that an individual can expect to lose will depend on many factors, including diet, exercise, and overall health. On average, individuals can expect to lose 1-2 pounds per week, but this can vary based on individual circumstances.

While exercise can help to burn calories and build lean muscle, diet plays a critical role in weight loss. It is important to choose a healthy diet that provides the body with all of the nutrients it needs to function properly and to avoid fad diets that may lead to yo-yo dieting and other health problems.

Finding a source of inspiration and setting achievable goals can help individuals to stay motivated during their weight loss journey. Additionally, choosing a form of exercise that is enjoyable and fitting with individual lifestyle and preferences can help to keep individuals on track and motivated.

Weight loss is an important issue that can bring about a wide range of benefits, including improved health, increased energy, and increased self-esteem. With the right approach, including a healthy diet, regular exercise, and a well-rounded weight loss plan, individuals can achieve their weight loss goals and improve overall health and wellness.

The journey to a healthier life and a healthy weight can be difficult and filled with obstacles. But with the right motivation and the right plan, you can find success and reach your goals. By understanding the problem with overweight, exploring different exercises and diet plans, and staying motivated throughout the process, you can make meaningful progress and work towards a healthier and lighter life.

The road ahead may be long and bumpy, but with the right dedication, you can make progress every single day. Don't be afraid to try something new, and don't forget to give yourself plenty of rest and relaxation. Most importantly, stay focused and motivated, and you'll find that you can make the necessary changes to live a healthier life and reach your weight loss goals. Good luck!

About the Author

Murali Dama is a highly accomplished individual with a diverse background in research and academia. He has completed a Ph.D. in Germany and followed it up with a postdoctoral research position in both Germany and the USA. He has an impressive publication record, with 16 articles in international journals, as well as experience reviewing articles and book chapters.

His research work focuses on food-related topics, and he has a wealth of knowledge on a variety of subjects including science, health, food, and more. He has worked in three different countries - India, Germany, and the USA - and worked with researchers from all over the world. His wealth of experience in both academia and research makes him an expert in his field. His knowledge on food, health, and science make him particularly well-suited to research and writing on these topics.